WHEN CANCER VISITS

How to Free Your Mind from the Grip of Distress and Heal Your Jolted Nervous System

by

Manuela M. Kogon, MD

DORRANCE
PUBLISHING CO
EST. 1920
PITTSBURGH, PENNSYLVANIA 15238

Dorrance Publishing Co
585 Alpha Drive
Pittsburgh, PA 15238
Visit our website at *www.dorrancebookstore.com*

ISBN: 979-8-88729-064-5
eISBN: 979-8-8872-9564-0

Cover art by Matthias Kogon

To my patients

I am awed by your integrity, wisdom, generosity, courage, and honesty.

If you find yourself described in this book, it might or might not be you.

To Matthias, Claudia, Peter, and Cristanne.

One life at a time.

To Ethan and Marty,

Thank You

ACKNOWLEDGMENTS

This is a big thank you to and great appreciation for my editor, Caroline Pincus. I was always intrigued reading the acknowledgments when cracking open a new book. Authors would write that their books would not have seen the light of day without their editor. I didn't really understand what that meant until I wrote one myself. This book would not have happened without Caroline.

When I first conceived the idea to try and convey to a larger audience what I do with individuals and groups, I had little experience in writing beyond an occasional science article. A friend introduced me to Caroline (thank you, Peter). When I presented her with my first draft, I don't remember her exact words, but she encouragingly stated that I had a good idea worth pursuing but also gently implied that my writing needed considerable work. She was right!

Caroline calls herself a book midwife. Her birthing assistance has been so expansive and transformative that I would probably call her a midwife *and* a doula. She not only helped deliver the baby, she accompanied the whole process almost from its inception, and as I discovered my writing voice, her feedback (even about the writing!) became more and more positive. Coming from a stock of literary people, including writers, publishers, bookshop owners, and book lovers, I was, for reasons still unclear to me, assigned to a math and science box in childhood. In hindsight this might have been a gift, as my doctor skills are what helped me find a place to express my love for language and words. And I hope the words have found their way into the hearts of cancer patients and their loved ones during a tremendously difficult time in their lives. Thank you, Caroline. Your experience, wit, knowledge, wisdom, depth, and humor have been invaluable. There most certainly wouldn't be a book to hold and cradle without you.

This is also a thank you to my son Ethan, who has an uncanny ability for diagonal reading and succinctly picking out idiosyncrasies in logic. "This doesn't make sense" was always a worth listening to encouragement to formulate better. I can't count the endless hours he spent on formatting and detecting inconsistencies in chaptering and content and gently guiding the stubborn mule into the digital age. With your skill set and personality, the world holds endless opportunities for you!

CONTENTS

PREFACE

Why You Might Want to Read This Book

Cancer sucks. I cannot change that. I can, however, help you smile. I can also help you take agency. I can help you to not freak out. I can help sharpen your thinking. I can help you sleep. And most importantly, I can help release the distress that comes with cancer that flavors every minute of your day. Whether you were just diagnosed with cancer, are cured from it, or have to live with it does not affect the help I can provide. In fact you do not even have to have cancer to profit from what is presented in this book. The global Covid-19 pandemic has jolted our nervous system. We all could use healing from the grip of distress.

Jacob had decided as a teenager that he would succeed no matter what. He dedicated his life to accomplishing goals he had set as a youngster. He did so with grit and determination. He frequently emphasized not being very smart and that he had accomplished everything in life with pure will. When he was diagnosed with cancer, he approached his illness very much the same way. Grinding down, not taking off from work during his treatment, never asking for rides to the hospital, for fear of—God forbid—inconveniencing anybody. As he became worn out as treatment was dragging on, his bravado persona started to crack. As is true for so many of his fellow cancer compadres, he realized that he had neglected other desires for too long. He had always very much enjoyed the companionship of his friends, especially outings with his old high school buddies for the last twenty-five years. But having focused on succeeding, he had forgotten how to enjoy leisure time.

He seemed relieved when I taught him the principle of competing and prioritizing needs.

"You mean I might be able to have both?" he asked. "Be successful *and* enjoy the companionship of my buddies?"

"Absolutely" was my answer as I guided him through the discovery of buried wishes and how to manage them. If you relate to Jacob, you will enjoy reading this book. I will walk you through the discovery or rediscovery of who you are and that you do not have to get lost in the emotional jungle of cancer.

When I first met Jacob, he casually mentioned that he had decided to follow the invitation of a friend to run a race together. Jacob's competitive self immediately checked the track record time in his age category and decided to beat it. After a couple of visits, however, he decided that his overruling need was companionship and enjoyment, not ambition. He ran the race with his friend who runs considerably more slowly than Jacob. I hope they both enjoyed it. Working with me will not turn you into a lazy slug. Working with me will help you become clear about who you are, what you want, and how to best turn your wishes into actions.

Needs and wants. At times we have to prioritize them, like Jacob, who always placed ambition over enjoyment. Sometimes we can have both, albeit not necessarily at the same time, but even that can be possible. With my coaching, Jacob figured out how to pursue his professional ambitions and reconnect to the things he most enjoyed in his life before cancer came visiting. **Chapter 8** is devoted to this idea of a need, want, and value-based life. To help prevent misunderstandings with language throughout the book, I want you to hear the meaning of the word "need" broadly, covering the range of options from absolute necessity (if I don't have it, I might die) to wants and likes (it would be nice to have this in my life). It's one of the chapters that stands on its own if you want to peek ahead.

Catherine had finished treatment for cancer. Everybody in her life was rejoicing and ready to resume their lives, but she sat in my office crying. Soon scheduled to go back to work, she could not fathom her reality.

"How can I go back to work as if nothing has happened? I have not even yet accepted that I have cancer," she pondered. She visibly relaxed and cracked a smile when I told her the story of the Sioux tribal member's maiden train ride. After deboarding at the first stop, he was seen sitting next to the tracks.

"What are you doing?" the departing passengers inquired.

"I am waiting for my soul to catch up," was his laconic answer.

If you are like Catherine, you know already that cancer adding itself uninvited to your life requires adjustment. Adjustment that will be different for different people. For Catherine it was about helping her soul "to catch up" to the shock of the diagnosis, let alone the treatment and its consequences. When you come to my office (or read this book), I help you identify if your soul needs to catch up to the shock of what is happening to you. I will help you identify what competing needs might hamper your life during the course of your illness. I will also show you how they can coexist. And I will enjoy harvesting the fruit of relief, joy, success, and delight with you.

People come to see me because their oncologist said, "Go see Kogon." When patients come "see Kogon" for their first visit, they usually expect the process to be something like talk therapy—what they associate with what a psychologist, counselor, or psychotherapist would do. Self-exploration, soul searching, expression of thoughts. My question about whether they keep their desk organized or enjoy breathing puzzles them, but when I deliver my recommendations to let their eyes rest on a tree or slowly exhale against the resistance of closed lips, together with an explanation of the physiology these recommendations are based on, most everybody is on board.

Spending time in nature makes intuitive sense, but hearing that you improve your focus and attention after a recent diagnosis of cancer by spending two hours a week in a natural outdoor environment will make you more readily look at that tree. Paying *voluntary* attention to the geometry of leaf patterns serves your health better than *involuntarily* paying attention to thoughts about funerals. As a cancer patient, it is in your best interest to be able to *voluntarily* pay attention to what matters rather than have your *involuntary* attention getting stuck on what feels most threatening and unmanageable.

When patients realize how liberating their discoveries can be, many even enjoy the process. Patients are intrigued when they notice that they can generate a change within themselves within minutes. You might feel lighter or less fatigued, lifting brain fog produces clearer thoughts and a shift in emotions eases you into a smile. It is a shift in experience that results in patients wanting to come back for more.

What I do is simple. I use the laws of biophysics and biochemistry to increase well-being. Like a martial arts master integrating the laws of gravity and leverage to effortlessly flatten an opponent, I'm inviting you to master the laws of thought and emotion to lighten your life. Cancer burdens your life. You will often hear me muse about the cost-benefit of behavior. I want to show you how to minimize behavior that adds burden and expand on behavior that adds ease. Improve the pleasure-to-distress ratio. Try to optimize pleasure and minimize distress. Every cell in your body will be grateful, be it a cell in your heart, brain, or liver.

What I do when people come see Kogon is help them balance their nervous system. Many of us, particularly where I teach and work, experience distress and its toll even without cancer. People often do not realize that their distress is affecting their emotions, mood, thinking, decision-making, motivation, and drive and that parts of the body signal this distress with insomnia, pain, irritability, and fatigue. Cancer, however, will jolt you out of complacency even if you were not distressed before.

Cancer leads to a fundamental paradigm shift. This can be quite upsetting. In my work, I help people ease this discomfort, often even turn it into joy and liberation. What I do is help people in the constant exchange of their experience with the world. A world that now has the word "cancer" omnipresent in it.

If you work with me (or read this book, which of course is also a way of working with me), you will learn why it is healthier to take a walk in the woods than downtown. If you work with me, you might have to stand on one leg while counting backwards from 100. Weird? Maybe. But effective. If you hear the physiology behind it, it will make perfect sense. Once you realize that the work brightens your thoughts, calms your heart, and lightens your body, you will be gung ho about taking control of your thoughts and emotions.

Is it scientific? Absolutely. Every action I teach you is based in the science of physiology. Nothing is ever "just because." Does it have a standardized protocol? Absolutely not. Every person is unique. Working with patients reminds me of dancing the tango. Leading effortlessly to create the perfect union. You will master the unconscious competence effortlessly when you are in the moment. No standardized protocol will ever teach you how to do that.

If you are a cancer patient, you probably have heard the term *targeted therapy or precision medicine*. This is what I do. I am the queen of *targeted precision medicine*—for the soul. What I do in my practice bewilders people at first.

"Is there a name for this?"

"Can I buy a book that teaches me?"

"No" to the first and absolutely "yes" to the second. You are holding it in your hand.

I have wondered if a book can replace a healing relationship. I'm not sure words on a page can adequately convey how I collaborate with patients, and I regret that. I often refer to these collaborations as dancing. But can the process that happens in an interaction be recreated by reading about it? My best hope is to come pretty close.

I hope that the many exercises in this book represent that process fairly well, so that it can benefit readers in a similar fashion to how patients benefit when working directly with me. You can read, practice, and share it with friends. I speculate that an important ingredient I contribute to the "growth-expediting process" is assistance in increasing self-awareness while reducing self-judgment. I know there is more involved, but I believe that these two components are core to easing personal growth. Let's continue to deepen our work on the path to healing.

The book is divided into a first part that addresses general principles of human physiology, anatomy, and biology, followed by parts devoted to cancer-specific issues. While you can go straight to the chapters that are most relevant to you, I urge you to read the introductory chapters, too, as they aim at understanding the basics of your functioning. With that understanding, desired change will be easier to achieve.

PREAMBLE

In this book, I am going to convince you that:

1) All we are is a heap of cells—a reasonably designed and coordinated heap of cells, but after all, just a heap of cells.
2) Misinformation about and misinterpretations of the function of these cells have led to many misconceptions of human functioning, leading to unnecessary suffering.
3) Having a better understanding of your personal heap of cells will allow you to experience greater well-being while going through the hell of cancer.
4) Looking at yourself as a heap of cells is liberating, as you will discover that the vast majority of your cells work just fine. Taking care of the minority, attention-seeking, unwelcome houseguests is manageable.

I remember vividly two books that lifted me onto the idea that something happens inside our body (or more precisely our brain) when we create a thought. It is hard to comprehend now that I could not grasp such a simple fact of biology. But it helps me understand patients who look at me blankly when I present them with the information. The books are so aptly titled *The Biology of Belief* by Bruce Lipton and *Molecules of Emotion* by Candace Pert. Both are beautifully crafted and humorously entertaining, the creators worthy of an invitation to an Iowa Writers Workshop.

"What? My brain cells have something to do with quantum physics?"

"What? There are serotonin receptors in my gut?" All of a sudden, I could relate to the fact that there is a physiological correlate to thought and emotion. In order for us to think and feel, electrical impulses get fired and chemical substances get produced and consumed. I suddenly became aware that I was a heap of cells.

I found it exquisitely liberating that cells are what are responsible for the generation of my thoughts and emotions. This discovery—that all of my experiences might be based in the physiology of my body and nothing else—both calmed and exhilarated me.

I hope that what I am presenting to you has the same effect on you.

INTRODUCTION

"Can you recommend a book?" is a question I am often asked by patients and healthcare providers alike. Much has been written about cancer. Books about the topic cover the whole range from scientific inquiry to self-help guide. Enter the word "cancer" into an Amazon search and fifty pages of cancer-related literature pop up. Do we need yet another book for search page fifty-one?

We have come a long way from cancer as death sentence to 70 percent of cancer patients living at least five years after diagnosis. Over 16 million cancer survivors live in the United States today, and there are estimates that the number will grow to almost 22.3 million by 2030. That's a lot of people. While there is still plenty of "slash, burn, and poison," as patients refer to their treatment, cancer treatment has made huge strides. Treatments have become more targeted to the cancer and individualized. Chemotherapy, surgery, and radiation are becoming elegantly sophisticated and innovative. As a society, we are speedily moving from "dying from cancer" to "living with cancer" when it comes to treatment.

The progress in cancer care has left many patients excited and searching. When it comes, however, to the emotional reaction and distress associated with cancer and how to best address these issues, society as a whole is lagging behind. This is also reflected in the literature available. There are more quality books about end-of-life issues than there are quality "cancer now" books. Patients have been dying from cancer for millennia, and the literature reflects the collected wisdom of centuries. It is surviving cancer and living with cancer that are new to humanity. People used to not "live with cancer." Now they do. I hope this book will add to the "cancer now" experience.

I have come across brilliant and eloquently written books about stress, communication, meditation, philosophy, health, positive psychology, and even cancer. But I have not encountered a book that effectively addresses stress and distress management for cancer patients and brings these different disciplines under one umbrella. A book that describes cancer patients' needs systemically and systematically from the time of diagnosis until after treatment and beyond. A book that also offers practical solutions to maintain some sense of normalcy and well-being while going through the experience of cancer. A book offering information about the physiology of that experience.

A book that a friend presses in your hand and says, "You have to read this."

Words are often not adequate to describe the experience of going through cancer (or many other things for that matter) and how to deal with it, but I hope I have come as close as possible to accompanying you through the experience with words.

This book is an attempt at encapsulating into words the work I do with individuals and groups, so it can reach a wider audience. It is also an attempt at translating the complexity of scientific knowledge into clinically practical exercises, which abates the terror of cancer and improves your well-being.

Cancer looms large. The National Cancer Institute estimates that 1,918,030 new cases of cancer will be diagnosed in the United States, and 609,360 people will die from the disease in 2022 alone. In 2019 there were an estimated 16,627,948 million people living with cancer in the United States. Worldwide there were 18.1 million new cancer diagnoses and 9.5 million cancer-related deaths in 2018. The number of new cancer cases is estimated to rise to 29.5 million by 2040.

At one point, I was hoping that this book could also serve to educate healthcare providers about the complexity of patients. Doctors' and patients' worlds, which are so intimately related during an experience with cancer, often seem far apart.

Misunderstandings, miscommunications, and disappointments complicate the already stressful mix of experiencing cancer. Patients and providers seem equally baffled by the metamorphosis that sometimes happens to patients' minds when their bodies undergo cancer. Not only is the experience confusing to patients, but to not have their doctors understand what they are going through compounds patients' bewilderment. But in trying to understand what my patients go through, I abandoned the wish to also write for doctors, as I found myself in a constant dance to please two audiences.

The book is intended to help patients not just to recognize but also solve problems that arise in the course of cancer. Patients and physicians after all share a goal, "Let's get the sucker!" or to be more biologically accurate, "Let's get the many tiny suckers that are trying to take over." If some doctors pick up the book in order to understand and empathize with their patients more deeply, even better.

Cancer is a complex illness with complex solutions requiring complex decisions. This book serves as much as a self-exploration tool for all of us as it serves as a self-exploration tool for people with cancer. Many aspects of human nature and human existence are universal. It is often just the setting in which we experience our humanness that differs. An emotional response to cancer can look very similar to a reaction to a car accident or the loss of your job. There are some universal components to human experience, and this book aims at presenting them in a comprehensible way.

Definitions of relevant words and core concepts are sprinkled throughout the book. They are purposely based on Google definitions because Google searches have become a standard source of knowledge for so many. The definitions are a good starting point of discussion and learning, even if they are not always accurate.

I decided to include them because I often witness people communicating without clarifying if they are talking about the same thing, and this often results in considerable distress and miscommunication. Defining is not just an aid to understanding yourself but also cardinal in creating a common denominator for communication and understanding with others. As you have probably experienced in your own—particularly intimate relationship—life, communication sometimes feels more like combative entrapment rather than illuminating enjoyment.

Learning is an interesting process. Do you remember times at school or college or even recently reading a newspaper article where you felt immediate frustration? Were you frustrated that your knowledge is too limited to grasp the extent or the depth of the information right away? Learning is a process. We cannot learn to ride a bike by hopping on it and expecting to enter an Olympic race. I want you to tolerate the process of learning. Learning is a spiral process of collecting pieces of information and revisiting them at a deeper level later. Educators describe the progression in learning as ascending from unconscious incompetence to conscious incompetence before you advance via conscious competence to unconscious competence as shown in Figure 1.

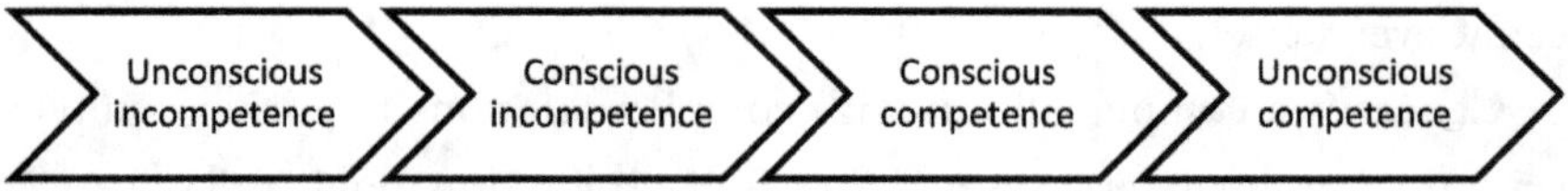

At times you will not grasp some content of this book right away. Lack of knowledge, experience, and practice will render you *un*consciously *in*competent. Simply read on as the information will be revisited. Knowledge consolidates in ways that does not always require actively thinking about it. Tango dancers know the pleasure of gliding across the floor with "unconscious competence." The brain knows how to consolidate information outside of conscious awareness! Let us learn!

PART I

CHAPTER 1.

Let's Get to Work

OUR FIRST AWARENESS EXERCISE

I believe in learning by experience. What can our heap of cells do? It can think, be content, and have bellyaches.

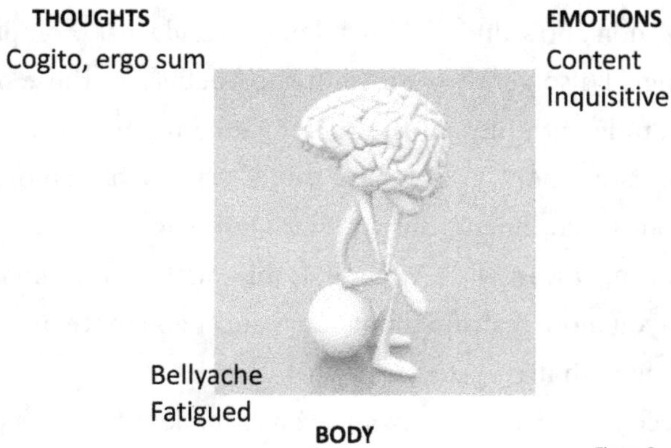

Figure 2

This particular heap of cells you see illustrated in Figure 2 was lying in bed on a sunny morning in 17th-century France. He was in ill health and felt fatigued and had a bellyache. Despite his physical ailments, he was content because he was inquisitive about his favorite activity: thinking. He was contemplating whether the mind was separate from the body. The thought of a disembodied mind. There is a hint in the picture about his identity. As a deep thinker, he was definitely "brain-heavy." The image reminds me of a self-reflection of a patient who calls herself a "brain on a stick."

His name is René Descartes. Ancient philosophers had contemplated the issue of mind before him, but the idea of separation of body and mind was named after him, the so-called Cartesian dualism. He held the opinion that mind was distinct from matter but could influence matter. Little did he know that centuries after his death, his ideas would still prevail. "Mind over matter" is a commonly used slogan. Mark Twain, always witty, knew how to use it.

"Age is an issue of mind over matter. If you don't mind, it doesn't matter."

Why am I introducing you to René Descartes? Because for cancer patients, Cartesian dualism is a particular problem. In our society, the idea of separation of mind and body is so ingrained that many patients have internalized the idea of "mind over matter." If not actually expecting to will their cancer away, patients often assume that if they just worked a little harder, they could at least have better control over their mind. They tell me that they "should think positive," they tell me that they "should not be stressed," they tell me that they "don't do sadness." While I understand what prompts patients to say these things, I also gently try to shift their beliefs, as those desires are often not compatible with physiology, thereby adding unnecessary distress. Reflecting on your situation, "matter over mind" is probably a more accurate expression of your predicament. Suspending Descartes' fascinating abstractions on rationalism, at least while you are dealing with your uninvited house guest, will make you more realistic about your cancer and more pragmatic and effective at dealing with it.

An early piece of advice comes from a cancer patient who was overheard saying at a treatment center in Santa Rosa, California, "I promise myself that I will never use the word "should" again" (Public eavesdropping clip in the *San Francisco Chronicle* reported on June 29, 2022).

When I first set out to write this book, I was convinced that mind only stems from matter, and mind is a production of body, mostly the brain. I have begun to consider that the mind might extend beyond the brain, but for the purpose of this book and its practical application, I'll stick to the idea that mind is matter. I am always happy to have a healthy philosophical argument, and I also do not want the spiritualists among you to turn away from this book, but I urge you to have an open mind about suspending Descartes' beliefs, at least temporarily, mostly to help you through cancer. Once you actually experience what your heap of cells is capable of, you will file Descartes' notion into the annals of philosophical thought for the next conversation with a friend or mentor.

Let's jump right into your personal experience with cancer and see how all this applies to how you can alleviate your discomfort. Take a moment to look at Figure 3 and describe yourself with the model I used for René Descartes. Start with paying attention to the process. Do you feel nervous about doing the exercise? Do you catch yourself in the thought about how stupid this exercise is and wonder how it can possibly help you? Are you pondering what an emotion is? Do you struggle sensing anything in your body? Or are you feverishly scribbling away, filling the lines? This is in fact your first awareness exercise. After reflecting on the process, pause to assess what you think right now, what you feel right now, and what you sense in your body right now, and jot it down on the lines or your smartphone.

THOUGHTS

....
....
....

EMOTIONS

....
....
....

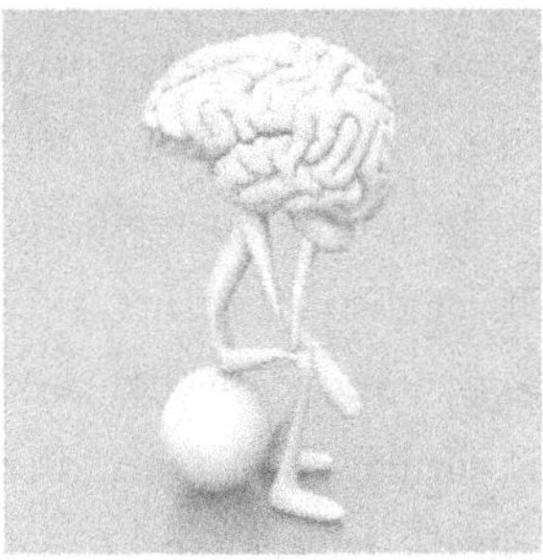

BODY ....
....
....

Figure 3

If you feel overwhelmed by the task, I have presented some options for you to pick from in Figure 4. If you are not in the mood to self-generate, circle what feels closest to your experience. It might jumpstart your own process. Thoughts, emotions, and physical sensations serve as window into ourselves and provide valuable clues to help us change.

Figure 4

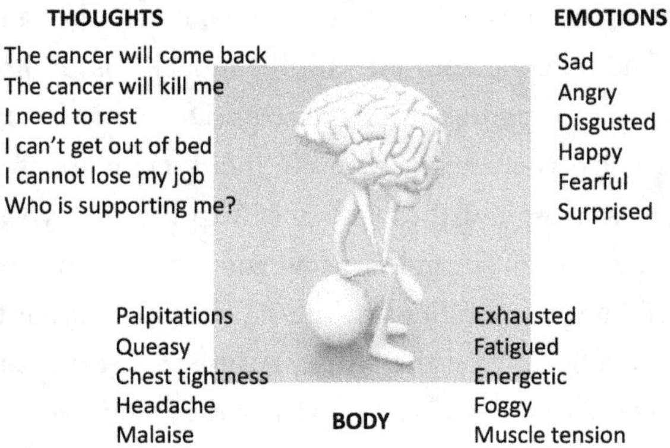

WE ARE ONE

I hope you are now on board with the differentiation of emotion, thought, and body you see in the picture. As you read on, I will try to convince you that emotion and thought are body generated, even if, like Descartes, many people think of thought and emotion in abstract terms. We refer to "Mind-Body" as two entities, but I'm going to convince you that they are one. Fortunately we are now seeing others making similar attempts at merging them back together in "integration." Three-hundred-fifty years of deviating from something that Aristotle knew all along! We are one. One big heap of cells.

I do not want to digress too far, but the following example is an illustration for statement two in the preamble (and it affects every patient): Misinformation about and misinterpretations of the function of our heap of these cells have led to many misconceptions of human functioning, leading to unnecessary suffering. Descartes' idea, Cartesian dualism, is deeply embedded in our health insurance system. Have you ever wondered why your health benefits have two aspects: "medical" benefits and "mental health" benefits? When our office coordinator tells me that I cannot see a particular patient because his or her mental health benefits are "carved out" from the insurance plan, I envision an ice cream scooper removing a dollop of brain mass. A memory emerges of me meticulously separating muscle fibers from each other with tweezers in the anatomy lab during medical school, the result resembling pulled pork. This particular part, which is carved out from the brain, is a second-class citizen with respect to reimbursement by insurance. "Body" reimbursements are usually more generous than "mind" or "mental" reimbursements.

And it is not just your benefits that take a hit. The separation of the brain into a mental and a physical part can have devastating consequences otherwise. Susannah Cahalan dedicates a whole book, *The Great Pretender*, to the problem. The author had ended up on a psych ward with an autoimmune disease of her brain that could've cost her her life until someone put two and two together and she received proper treatment.

As a cancer patient, this is important as many of your distress-related symptoms get misinterpreted as psychiatric problems. In the next section, **You Are Not Crazy,** I will provide the evidence to make sure you will recognize your symptoms accurately and not share Cahalan's fate.

I understand why people struggle with "physical" versus "non-physical," and I want to illustrate by paraphrasing a post from one of the webinars I help teach. A student posted "when you go beyond the physical, which is the visible, you get the emotional and psychological aspects of pain which, if left unaddressed, can mean that treatment may be less effective."

It is much easier to relate to physical pain, such as pain in the foot or the neck because you can touch it and point at it. People don't think of emotional pain, such as sadness or despair, in the same way. You cannot touch the part in the brain that is involved in creating the experience "despair," thus I understand my student's reference to visibility.

I am intrigued by the notion that the invisibility of emotions would leave them more likely to go unaddressed. The student is right. Those aspects of cancer care (or any other illness) get addressed less. But by no means are they invisible.

In this day and age of neuroscience, that statement is not based in science but in Cartesian dualism. You can see distress on a heart rate variability monitor as easily as you can see a broken foot on an x-ray. Do not treat pain in the foot differently from despair in the brain. Not just are we ONE, as coordinated as possible, heap of cells, all cells follow the same laws of biophysics and biochemistry, regardless of whether the cells fire from the toe or the brain.

Not fully understanding the body and its function opens the door to misunderstandings and actions based on erroneous beliefs. If you believe that the generation of emotions is under the control of will, you are more likely to come to the conclusion that you should not feel a certain way. And you are more likely to be annoyed if your body generates the emotion anyway regardless of your belief. But if you know that what you feel is a spontaneous generation of your body, you have numerous options to act in your body's interest once the emotion is generated. Even if you cannot touch an emotion and see it like a broken toe. In this day and age of neuroscience, the presumably intangible has become tangible.

I understand people's desire to think in categories. There is nothing wrong with wanting to create a category of mental health disorders, per se. For centuries we had no understanding of the brain other than observation of its action. And so humans filled the mystery with an abstract concept. Understandable. I can even understand why these concepts are kept in place to defend interests. But it is hard to understand why not more people question the paradigm and why we would base that categorization on a philosophical idea rather than anatomy and science. The equivalent would be building a self-driven car with 200-year-old technology. Don't you want the latest knowledge to be the basis for building the car?

This aspect of categorization is particularly important for cancer patients who often find themselves diagnosed with a mental health diagnosis they do not have. The mental health diagnosis will add insult to injury to an already-distressed mind. The distress that is part of cancer does not merit a mental health diagnosis (This of course does not mean that a mental health diagnosis cannot coexist or preexist or develop as part of cancer).

"Humankind cannot bear much reality." This quote from T.S. Eliot is very much aligned with that notion. We like to "know," and if we don't "know," we tend to fill the gaps by simply making things up and call it reality. We simplify. We categorize. We spiritualize. In medicine simplification can be a problem. Categorizations do not describe physical reality. They describe models and approximations of reality. Do not allow that to happen to you.

I was delighted to learn about Professor Andrew McIntosh, chair of biological psychiatry at the University of Edinburgh, who said, "We hope our research will encourage people to think ...whether physical and mental illnesses are as separate as some believe," when reporting his finding that an individual with a partner or spouse who has chronic pain has a higher risk of chronic pain themselves (McIntosh et al., 2016). Now that is an example of mind-body connection! To the mind and body of the person next to you!

And I felt optimism when I learned that David Ross from Yale University is leading an initiative to integrate neuroscience into psychiatry residency curricula. At the time of starting to write this book, less than half of psychiatry training programs in the U.S. had formal neuroscience teaching with a neuroscientist on staff. I am looking forward to the day when neurology and psychiatry will be reunited (they used to be one) in one specialty again.

YOU ARE NOT CRAZY

Studies examining the prevalence of mental health disorders in cancer patients show that most cancer patients do not meet the diagnostic criteria for any specific mental disorder (Derogatis et al., 1983, Massie & Holland, 1987). If the majority of people don't have a psychiatric diagnosis, we shouldn't use a psychiatric diagnostic system to categorize them. But that does not mean we should ignore patients' emotional needs and problems.

Assessing patients' needs and discomfort is key, but it must not lead to patients feeling that their symptoms constitute a psychiatric problem. Pathologizing an experience can be traumatic in itself. Having "Major Depression" is very different from having depressive symptoms. The prevalence of what we conventionally call depression and anxiety is similar in patients with cancer compared to the general population. Thus using standard diagnostic tools to assess depression and anxiety will not help differentiate the cancer patients from the general population with respect to their relevant problems. If you want to know what bugs cancer patients, you have to use different assessment tools.

A prodigious data review analyzed by Mitchell and collaborators was published in *Lancet Oncology* in 2013. They compared over 50,000 cancer patients and over 200,000 physically healthy people with respect to depression and anxiety. 11.6 percent of cancer patients versus 10.2 percent of the healthy control had depression. Even in such a large sample, that is not considered a statistical difference. The data for anxiety were slightly different. 18 percent of cancer patients reported anxiety, and 14 percent of the healthy people reported anxiety. Saying that eighteen versus fourteen people out of 100 people feel anxious doesn't seem that much of a difference; statistically, however, that is considered a real difference due to the large sample size. Clinically it makes sense.

Cancer patients are not mentally sick, but the activation of their nervous system due to distress can easily mimic mental illness. I will discuss how what encompasses "anxiety" is mostly driven by what happens to us when the nervous system gets activated and starts messing with the brain. The activation of the nervous system results in distress that can make getting cancer feel similar to what veterans experienced after getting back from a military tour in Afghanistan or Iraq. Addressing that distress is crucial.

WHY DO I FEEL SO WEIRD?

What I am trying to do here is look at the experience of cancer—at what we experience when we are diagnosed with cancer and go through treatment and beyond—through the lens of stress and distress and also differentiate them from each other. At no point do I ever want anyone to walk away with the idea that distress *causes* cancer. I find myself counseling people on this point all the time. This kind of thinking is too simplistic and causes much suffering. Development of cancer is intricately complex.

The important distinction here is that yes, distress affects your health, but cancer is not your fault. And distress can certainly exacerbate symptoms that are accompanying cancer, such as pain, insomnia, cognitive difficulty, and fear among others. But you did not *cause* your cancer. One of my goals here, in fact, is to integrate cancer supportive care into cancer care rather than cart it off to psychiatric care. Unfortunately this is currently not the predominant approach!

The National Comprehensive Cancer Network, an alliance of leading cancer centers, suggests that we in cancer care use the term "distress" rather than "psychiatric, psychosocial, or emotional disorders," as it is less stigmatizing and embarrassing. The terminology helps normalize the mental health aspects of an already stressful experience. I am very much on board with that. And that's why I offer you solutions to "de-stress" away from "distress." For one simple reason: When we de-stress, many of our physical functions work better, as you soon will learn.

There is increasing interest in the assessment of distress and its detrimental impact on health. Blood pressure, pulse, temperature, and breathing rate are already used in every standard health assessment. There is some movement to add the assessment of distress to the basic set of what are called vital signs. A short questionnaire assesses not just distress related to emotional and physical problems but inquires about other sources of distress, such as family, practical, and spiritual concerns. If the cause of your distress is financial, sending you to a psychiatrist will accomplish little but connecting you with a social worker can do wonders.

Several studies have investigated the prevalence of distress as measured by the National Comprehensive Cancer Network Distress Thermometer (DT) (Carlson et al., 2012). While there is a range among the different studies, most everybody is in agreement that a majority of cancer patients are in distress.

When reading Linda Carlson's article, I rejoiced reading that "Distress is not a precise clinical term that appears in the Diagnostic and Statistical Manual of Mental Disorders, Fourth Edition, which is used to assign formal psychiatric diagnoses, but it is part of the clinical significance criterion that is a qualifier for several mood disorders, including major depression and adjustment disorder.

One reason for its adoption in cancer care is that the term distress is often more useful for cancer clinicians than psychiatric terms, such as anxiety or depression." What a relief. I am not the only one thinking along these lines!

In this book, I treat all of your cells equally. I do not treat "mind" cells differently from "body" cells. The cells in the tip of your nose have similar core functions as the brain cells that generate feelings. In illness we often focus on what does not work instead of expanding what does work. As I mentioned earlier, I want to help you realize that many of your cells are doing their job just fine. We will only treat the cells that need it.

OUR SECOND AWARENESS EXERCISE

Let us implement these thoughts into another exercise. The first exercise was about assessing what is. Let us add an exercise to discover what is well. To get practice, let us start with the first exercise again. If you are someone who prefers to listen over reading the instruction, create or have a friend create an audio version of the following instructions you can then listen to.

Take a moment to focus on your thoughts and mentally record consecutive thoughts as if you were recording them on your handheld device. Then make the same assessment with your emotions. Can you identify them? Then move on to your physical sensations. Do you have any body sensations, and what are they? Take your time to make this assessment. And always make sure to take a breath that focuses on slowly exhaling in between every assessment. The simple action of breathing signals information to the brain to balance the nervous system. If you struggle taking deep breaths or are self-conscious about "breathing right," simply record thought, emotion, and body sensation without especially paying attention to breath.

As you are doing the exercise, observe what makes you unique. Are you one of those people who generate 50,000 thoughts a day? Are you someone who thinks more unhappy thoughts than happy thoughts? Are you someone whose thoughts seem to have a life of their own and seem to fire beyond the grasp of your control? Are you someone who does not quite know what an emotion feels like? Or are you someone who has so many emotions that at times you feel like you are drowning in them? Or maybe your emotions oscillate like ocean swells? Or do you have plenty of physical experiences but don't know whether to attribute them to cancer or a harmless cold?

As you are now in the process of assessing what is good or bad, pleasant or uncomfortable, let us turn our attention towards what works well. Take a moment to scan your body for the possibility of one cell that feels good. And if most of your cells feel shitty, maybe you can find one cell that feels at least alright. Can you conjure up the image of a cell? Your image does not have to be based in real-life biology. You can simply imagine a round circle, plump and juicy. And don't feel discouraged if you have a hard time creating images. Look in a book or online at what a cell looks like and use the image for this exercise.

Can you find a place in your body where such a cell exists? Maybe the tip of your nose, maybe a cell in your left thumb, or could it be a cell in your right toe? Simply take a moment to scan your body for such a cell. Don't fret if you don't make the connection, I promise that by the end of the book you will.

If you have identified a healthy cell somewhere in your body, take a moment to look at what you see with your mental eye. A round, plump, healthy cell? Or does your mind create a different image? Do you feel courageous enough to expand from where you are now and look at the cell next to this one healthy cell? Remember we have trillions and trillions of them. What does the cell next to the healthy cell look like? Simply let your mind play with the idea.

In a last step, observe whether your sense of comfort or discomfort changed during the exercise. Do you feel better? Do you feel worse? And if you feel different, how? Have your thoughts taken on a different quality? Has an emotion shifted? Or has a body sensation changed?

MEET MR. BALDWIN

Going forward I want you to internalize the following image. Figure 5 presents us with the notion that the external world and our internal world are in a constant back-and-forth exchange. Like playing a round of table tennis.

Figure 5 is an expansion of Figure 3 and 4. We assessed that our internal world is composed among other things of thoughts, emotions, and body sensations. But now we are adding what happens in our exchange with the external world. As the picture depicts, a car cutting you off might make you think about your fear and might make your heart beat faster.

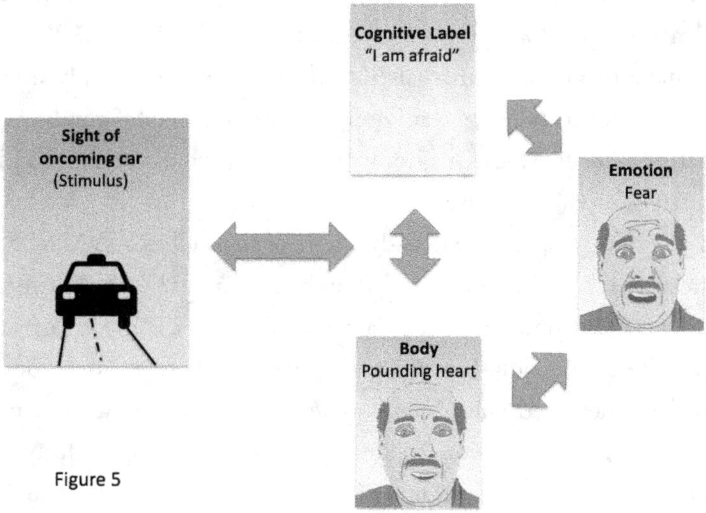

Figure 5

As the picture presents, those entities are in an internal ping-pong with each other as well. You thinking about your fear will contribute to making your heart beat faster, not just the car driving at you. This image is going to be a roadmap that accompanies you throughout the book. I want you to internalize the image and to be able to pull it up from memory.

You can create your own personal version or download one from the Internet also. If you don't want to be a bald guy, make him prettier. Many of the exercises in this book contain components of what you see in the picture. As you continue reading, you will go into more depth about these individual components of thought, emotion, and body. An important purpose of the first two exercises to assess your own experience was to familiarize you with the basic idea.

SALUTOGENESIS

As the exercise prompted, my aim here is to encourage you to focus on your health and not just your illness. The illness itself naturally will demand much attention on various levels, but you don't have to let it become all-consuming.

Focusing on your health is a great counterbalance. "Salutogenesis" (*salus* means health or safety in Latin, and *genesis* is the Greek word for origin, creation, and generation) is a term coined by Aaron Antonovsky, a Yale-trained academic. It describes an approach that focuses on attending to factors that facilitate health and well-being rather than factors that cause disease (pathogenesis). Antonovsky was researching the health of Holocaust survivors and found that one in three holocaust survivors was emotionally and physically healthy compared to 50 percent of the general population.

Rather than focusing on the causes to explain the difference, which seemed a no-brainer to him, given the horrors they had gone through, he was contemplating what made it possible for one out of three people to stay healthy despite the barbarity they had endured.

His research distilled three factors—manageability, comprehensibility, and meaningfulness—as important ingredients for health. I am not sure how anybody in a concentration camp could have a sense of manageability and comprehend anything and find meaning, but there seems to be something about those factors that helped people survive.

I observe that the lack of these three entities is, at times, what propels cancer patients into a state of frenzy and despair. All of a sudden, your life does not feel manageable, and it is very hard to comprehend why you even got cancer to begin with. Meaning can become a core feature patients reflect on as well.

The same way Mr. Baldwin gives you company throughout the book, Antonovsky's research illustrates a principle that will accompany you as well, which is the idea of core needs. Antonovsky used the expression to create a "sense of coherence." Coherence, like stress, is a term borrowed from physics to refer to waves having the same frequency. I think of it as being in sync. Our needs have to be in sync with each other.

As you have learned from Mr. Baldwin's ping-pong, it is not just about what happens in the outside world but how we perceive events in our surroundings. Not having important needs, such as manageability or comprehension or meaning met, can be quite disturbing to your system. Those three needs are just part of a pool of options.

Always keep in mind your individuality, which I have pointed out from the get-go. Your personal core needs might be different, as we will explore in **Chapter 8** on **The Concept of Human Needs**. You can take some time and explore this now, before resuming reading, if you want to practice and deepen your understanding of yourself. As I have mentioned, learning is not always linear.

Focusing on something other than her illness is something the esteemed author Winnifred Gallagher succinctly described in her book *Rapt: Attention and the Focused Life*. In line with Mr. Baldwin's exchange with the world, she explores the idea that what we pay attention to very much flavors what we experience, not just what happens on the outside. Winifred Gallagher described that "after the biopsy from hell," she intuited that "this disease wanted to monopolize my attention, but as much as possible, I would focus on my life instead." This is very much aligned with the idea of focusing on things other than cancer. It does not always have to be focusing on health only but on anything that helps you not get consumed by cancer, figuratively and literally speaking.

WHAT IS MIND?

In order to execute the wellness awareness exercise you just did, you had to engage your mind. As I steer you away from the idea that you have a "mental disorder," I do not intend to steer you away from "mental" or "mind." Let's get the conversation about mind out of the way so you are not constantly wondering "what is mind exactly?" while you are reading.

We tend to use the word very casually. Have you ever thought about what "mind" is? Take a moment to reflect on your own definition. I already made you work hard on the first few pages of the book, so why not engage your mind a little more?

Presumably you just spent a minute or so on a definition of "mind." Daniel Siegel, a researcher at UCLA, has spent a lifetime studying the subject. In his book *Mindsight*, he describes how he came to define the mind. It was the result of a several year-long interdisciplinary group collaboration of over forty scientists coming from a broad range of fields, including philosophy, computer science, genetics, sociology, neuroscience, and psychology. They were trying to tackle the question of whether the physical nature of the brain is related to the subjective nature of the mind. Depending on their specialties, the scientists came up with very different definitions.

After much contemplation, the group settled on the following: "The human mind is a relational and embodied process that regulates the flow of energy and information." Whatever your personal opinion about this definition and whatever your beliefs, I think we are all in agreement that if part of "matter," part of the heap of cells, develop a life of their own, a.k.a. become cancerous, the "mind" will have its work carved out, regardless of whether you think that mind is just the "activity of the brain" or the mind "constitutes our thoughts and feelings" or is a "shared social process passed across the generations," just to quote a few definitions the group of scientists around Dan Siegel were debating.

"The human mind is a relational and embodied process that regulates the flow of energy and information" leaves a lot of room for your own thinking. This definition is an inspiration for reflecting on who you are. Knowing that "mind" is fundamental to the creature "human." And fundamentally affecting and contributing to a human with cancer.

NEUROPLASTICITY

The same way you need an understanding of "mind" to grasp the content of this book, understanding "neuroplasticity" will be beneficial also. Neuroplasticity refers to the ability of the heap of brain cells to change.

Many exercises in this book are based on neuroplasticity. We take advantage of the fact that the brain is malleable.

When I went to medical school, I was taught that the brain is a static entity whose function is set at birth. You had to live with what you got. Talk about "misinformation and misinterpretations leading to misconceptions" as I had expressed with preamble two. The brain is not static at all. It is a lively, constantly adapting and changing heap of cells.

My introduction to the topic was a book by Sharon Begley, *Train Your Mind, Change Your Brain*. I was immediately enthralled by the idea that my brain might not just be an inert lump with all its associated fallibilities I thought I had to live with. There was evidence that I could change it. In recent years, many books have followed to present the evidence. One of my favorites is *The Brain's Way of Healing* by Norman Doidge. Many suggestions in my book are based on the assumption that nerve cells can grow the same way muscle fibers can.

I often advise my patients to imagine going to a gym for brain training and grow their brain cells the same way they grow their muscle cells. Lifting weights make muscles grow, engaging brain cells makes brains grow.

Siegrid Löwel wrote in a scientific article, "Neurons wire together if they fire together." That has morphed into the popular neuroscience saying, "Neurons that fire together wire together." If we can grow cells, we can also shrink the parts we don't want. When you engaged in awareness exercise one and two, you started changing your brain. Numerous exercises throughout the book will help you mold your brain into what suits you best.

So how can we best use our heap of cells? Consider that what you have learned in your life about the mind may not be serving you well. If you believe, as I did, that the brain is a fixed entity or that energy medicine is "bogus," then you risk closing off numerous avenues to catalyze health. If you are receptive to the principles of neuroplasticity, you open paths to take better control of thoughts and emotions.

We are supposed to use our cells to the best of our ability. Descartes definitely did. He was a brilliant philosopher, scientist, and mathematician. I cannot fault the poor man that his ideas got applied to the wrong situation. To best use your heap of cells, you have to stay sharp and informed and assemble a supportive team around you.

WHEN WE ARE STUPID, WE ARE STUPID

In order to help anchor some of the information I want you to retain, let me talk about a few scientists, their lives, and their discoveries. The scientists' lives and research moved me deeply because of their integrity and determination not to give up on their beliefs and hypotheses about how things work, which often only much later proved to be true or become accepted. And they are very much relevant to the practice of medicine today.

The primatologist Frans de Waal, in his eloquently and entertainingly written book, *Are We Smart Enough to Know How Smart Animals Are?*, does a wonderful job of pointing out human limitations with respect to observational skills and interpretations. His expertise is in the animal world but very much applies to the cancer world. I did not want to get myself into trouble with my colleagues by calling my book *Are Health Care Providers Smart Enough to Know How Smart Cancer Patients Are?* but the question would be relevant, raising important issues in cancer care.

I often witness cancer patients making astute and insightful observations about themselves and their circumstances. Sadly the providers giving them care, out of a combination mostly of inexperience and lack of awareness, can be limited in their ability to relate. What results are often unnecessarily hurtful interactions between patients and providers.

I am mostly okay (most of the time) being a speck in the universe, but sometimes I detect a tinge of envy that I could not be the one who said, "We must remember that what we observe is not nature itself, but nature exposed to our methods of questioning." De Waal uses the quote by the German physicist Werner Heisenberg to illustrate that long-held erroneous beliefs by scientists about animals were related to experiments that were not set up intelligently to capture what the scientists actually wanted to measure. I picked one example from his to illustrate the importance of staying aware that how we look at nature, which includes how we look at ourselves, has limitations with respect to truly seeing how we are. That has the potential to get us in trouble. If you are undergoing chemotherapy and are looking for reading material, you can enjoy de Waal's illuminating book during your infusions. I think it will make you laugh and question yourself in a good way. Laughter is good for your health, right (Mora-Ripoll, 2010)? And more importantly: its benefits were also examined in cancer patients (Kim et al., 2015).

De Waal drives home his point with an example. At one point, someone decided that elephants are dumb based on an experiment that previously had yielded interesting data for monkeys. The ability to use tools was the measurement of animal intelligence. Researchers left a stick under a palm tree. Monkeys would take the stick and bang down the bananas. Elephants did not. Ergo: elephants are dumb.

Fortunately someone figured out that elephants did not pick up the stick because it would block their nasal passages, and with the obstruction, they could not smell. Again fortunately someone thought to set up the experiment more intelligently. They placed a box near the tree. Sure enough the elephant stepped on it and grabbed the bananas off the tree. Elephants would even retrieve a box that was hidden someplace else and push it toward the tree. So who is dumb? Elephants or humans?

This particular example moved me as I recently read an article in the newspaper describing how elephants in Kenya seem to have developed a sense for where poachers loom. The elephants move either to the borders of the reserve where there are fewer poachers or close to ranger stations to protect themselves as a herd. As a cancer patient, you often don't get the most effective tools to manage your distress. Make sure to seek the tools that get you the bananas.

COGNITIVE BIAS

I have plenty of my own "Heisenberg" moments. I love to swim. For most of my life, that meant swimming in a pool. I was never surprised when my bathing suits disintegrated after a while. That was part of swimming. A few years ago, I discovered swimming in the ocean. What is going on with my bathing suits? They have stayed intact for years. Instead of buying five suits a year, I buy one! Then it finally dawned on me. The dissolving of fabric had nothing to do with the water or swimming. It was the chlorine in the pool! I had to remember that "what we observe is not nature itself but nature exposed to our methods of questioning." My own methods of questioning in this particular example were obviously not very foolproof.

This is a silly example, I know, but it highlights that we have to be aware of our cognitive limitations. Check in with yourself for times when you were either ignorant or unobservant until some factor later emerged that changed your perception of the situation and you found yourself feeling stupid for your earlier ignorance. There are many ways that our thinking ends up becoming faulty, and it is fundamental to know some principles so we can overcome some of them through training.

The example I gave illustrates what is called "attribution error." The term is usually used to describes humans' tendency to attribute people's behavior to their disposition and underestimate the importance of situation. For instance Mr. Baldwin being cut off by a car is likely to think the driver is a rude idiot, but perhaps the driver was rushing to visit his sick wife in the hospital and accidentally cut off Mr. Baldwin in his fearful hurry. Context is important.

We are basically creating our own reality to suit all kind of purposes. If you have cancer, that is a problem as you don't want your biases to influence your decision-making.

Humans also have a tendency for what is called "confirmation bias." We tend to interpret evidence as confirmation of our existing beliefs rather than consider evidence that would disprove it. There are numerous illustrations in the research literature, but our minds default to rationalize rather than to be rational.

Imagine you make a conscious effort to look for balanced information about a surgical procedure, but your confirmation bias trips you up and you end up looking only for data with a good outcome. You will not be objective in evaluating the cons of your choices. We see what we want to see and not necessarily what is there.

As a cancer patient, it is fundamental that you are as close to your biological reality as possible, in part to choose the best treatment options. If you understand your biology and physiology, it will also help greatly to decrease distress while sick. At the beginning of this book, I said that what I do is simple. That I use the laws of biophysics and biochemistry to design simple interventions to improve well-being. Understanding the laws of confirmation bias will help you feel less stupid about your ignorance. It is a natural part of who we are. Acknowledging the existence of bias will help you search for the cues to decrease your cognitive illusions. In later chapters, you will get to work on your biases and practice not just to detect them but decrease them.

THE SCIENCE OF TODAY IS THE ERROR OF TOMORROW

It is not just our bias that leads us astray. Jakob Johann Baron von Uexküll, another brilliant mind, described that "Die Wissenschaft von heute ist der Irrtum von morgen" (The science of today is the error of tomorrow). Think about that for a moment. For a long time, no one questioned that the earth was flat. That seems ridiculous now, but there is an example from the cancer world to demonstrate his point.

For many years women were prescribed estrogen as hormonal replacement therapy (HRT). It eased symptoms during menopause considerably. That was a plus, and it was standard of care. But only because we did not know any better. A collaborative effort analyzing data revealed in the 1990s that the practice had a considerable risk. The inquiry was published in the preeminent medical journal *Lancet*. The risk of getting breast and uterine cancer was considerably higher when using HRT.

If an article makes it into *Lancet*, people, pay attention! But please do not misinterpret this later research either. Hormone replacement does not cause cancer. It comes with a higher risk of cancer, but this does not mean you automatically get cancer when you use it. There are situations in medicine when we still use it and should.

There is another situation that makes the news for which we do not know "nature" yet. It has to do with whether or not talcum powder causes ovarian cancer. When you interview women who are sick with ovarian cancer, it appears that more of these women used talcum powder in the past than women who do not have ovarian cancer. However, when we compare all women using talcum powder with women who do not, there does not seem to be a difference with respect to developing more ovarian cancer (Wentzensen & O'Brien, 2021).

The latter, by the way, is what is called a "prospective study," meaning you are comparing two groups (in this case, a group using talcum powder versus one not using talcum powder to see if they have different outcomes at a later point, e.g. development of cancer).

If you want to dive straight into the pitfalls of statistics and its meaning for individuals, you can peek at the section on **Dealing With Statistics** in **Chapter 11**.

Statistics can be very confusing, but don't give up on them. I'm going to show you how not to throw in the towel when it comes to dealing with statistics. As a cancer patient, there is no way to avoid them as many of your decisions are and will be based on statistical probabilities.

STANDARD OF CARE IS NOT ALWAYS BEST CARE

As we've seen, sometimes we err and adjust when we learn that we are wrong. Sometimes we continue to do wrong, even where there is good evidence that we should not. History is full of stories about scientists who were correct in their observations but were rejected by their peers at the time. Can you imagine that at one point doctors washing their hands before touching you was not standard of care? Thousands of women during childbirth found out the hard way. Not doing so cost millions of lives, including the one of the people who first advocated doing so. He was way ahead of his time.

Ignaz Semmelweis, a Hungarian physician in the 19th century, realized that childbed fever had something to do with lack of hygiene on the part of the doctors. Puerperal fever as it was also known was common and often fatal. Semmelweis was able to reduce mothers' mortality dramatically by simply washing his hands before assisting with birth.

His breakthrough observations in 1847 conflicted with the echelons of the scientific establishment in Vienna, where he was practicing at a hospital. Physicians were offended at the suggestion to wash their hands. Semmelweis could offer no scientific explanation for his findings. He operated purely on clinical observations. His story ended tragically. Trying to convince the medical establishment unsuccessfully, his increasingly bitter rants earned him a trip to the lunatic asylum in 1865, where he died within fourteen days of admission.

If scientists had been a little swifter in recognizing a brilliant mind, it would have even saved the life of the 20th president of the United States. It was not the bullets that killed James A. Garfield when he was shot on July 2nd, 1881. They had securely lodged in the president's abdomen without doing deadly damage. It was the physicians digging around with their dirty hands to remove them that caused the president to die eleven weeks later on September 19th, 1881, riddled with abscesses all over his body. Even more tragic than Semmelweis' knowledge not having made it across the pond was the fact that antiseptic practice was widely used in England and had been introduced to American physicians already in 1876 after a visit from the British antiseptic advocate Joseph Lister.

But ignorance is not limited to the 19th century. Barry Marshall's story has at least a happy outcome. He won the Nobel Prize. But he took quite a risk to get there. Like myself Dr. Marshall had learned in medical school that ulcers of the stomach were related to stress, too much acid and spicy food. In the 1980s, he hypothesized that a bacterium called H. pylori might be involved in the process of developing stomach ulcers. The medical establishment was not supportive of Dr. Marshall's hypothesis. No one could imagine that bacteria could live in a very acidic environment. To prove his point, Dr. Marshall swallowed a petri dish of H. pylori bacteria and got violently sick with gastritis. He had made his point.

Bennet Omalu's story is still ongoing. The intelligent doctor from Nigeria lived the American dream. After his medical education in Africa, he moved to Pittsburgh to work as a pathologist, getting two Masters degrees on the side. He knew nothing about football, but he discovered that repetitious concussions can have damaging consequences to the brain. Many football players had exhibited symptoms after their retirement without realizing the nexus.

Omalu could not fathom why the NFL did not welcome him with open arms to learn from his discoveries and protect their players. It took the NFL several years before they publicly acknowledged the problem and even longer before they did anything about it. Dr. Omalu's scientific and human integrity has been very inspiring to me. But following his story, I don't know if he personally thinks it was worth the price he and his wife paid, having to move the family across the country to start over personally and professionally.

WHO DO I TRUST?

Are you wondering why I am using examples to illustrate medical shortcomings of past and present? My intent is not to cultivate doubt in medicine but to inspire you to expand your awareness. In your journey with cancer, you have yourself and your knowledge that you have accumulated over time to draw from in your attempt at optimizing your health, and you have collective knowledge accumulated over centuries. When you are diagnosed with cancer, that moment in time constitutes one point on your life continuum embedded in the ocean of many continuums. The more aware and knowledgeable you are about yourself, the more likely you will be able to distill from the vast and endless ocean of contemporary available knowledge what is relevant to you and to find the right people to help you with it. **Chapter 11** on **Dealing With Diagnosis** will walk you through the details of how to find them.

As a patient, it is a tight rope to walk. You can try to optimize yourself and optimize your surroundings. But the decision to learn about yourself and learn from the collective knowledge that might pertain to your illness is not always easy. Whether to participate in your care or whether to surrender and simply trust that someone will make the best choices for you is a balancing act and a set of choices that is different for every individual.

What if you are treated by contemporary medical cutting-edge knowledge that later turns out to be wrong, or you are treated by someone ridiculed as a hogwash quack who later turns out to be right? We cannot walk around wondering constantly about the veracity of current opinion. Sometimes we just have to trust an expert. No cancer patient can acquire adequate knowledge in time to make a truly informed decision. This naturally evokes fear and insecurity. The best you can do is assemble a team of people that you believe do the best they can within their area of expertise.

It can be so daunting to make challenging decisions about your own life. For physicians to help you make these challenging decisions is also daunting. You want your doctors to do the best they can without feeling stifled by the possibility of making a mistake. You also want them to have the courage to sometimes make an unorthodox decision because their life exposure or clinical experience tells them that they are right. Sometimes we have to follow convention to make an impact; sometimes we have to be the lone ranger in the desert making a non-conforming decision to save a life. That is true for patients and doctors alike.

THE ABSENCE OF EVIDENCE IS NOT THE EVIDENCE OF ABSENCE

What can we learn from the errors of the past? Can we use our heap of cells to minimize the chance of error for our own future and the future of others? If we are a machine with all these kinks, we have to make accommodation for the kinks or at least be thoughtful about their existence. Otherwise the malfunctioning of our machine becomes an obstacle.

As a cancer patient, you have incredibly difficult choices to make, and as physicians, we have incredibly difficult choices to present. "The absence of evidence is not the evidence of absence" reminds us that just because we do not know or understand does not mean something does not exist.

I encourage your heap of cells to stay open-minded and curious. I want you to be open to consider that you are wrong, even if you think you are right, and consider being right even if someone else thinks you are wrong. And sometimes it's not about right or wrong in any objective sense. Anything is possible. Human experience and its individual idiosyncrasies cover a wide range on a continuum of possibilities. You place somewhere on that continuum with your uniqueness. So let's make sure that we serve you as best as we can for whatever you need.

I don't want to leave you the impression that science, including medicine, is stumbling through the centuries making accidental discoveries and constant mistakes. Individuals with devotion, intelligence, passion, and drive have contributed wonderful things to the accumulated collective knowledge. We evolve as individuals and we evolve as a society. History has collected a vast ocean of information that we can all benefit from if we look for it without getting lost in it.

THE CONTINUUM OF HUMAN EXISTENCE AND THE PLEASURE OF STATISTICS

We learned how Aaron Antonovsky encourages us to focus on health rather than illness. His work represents another principle that will be important to you and your health. Antonovsky rejected the dichotomy of health versus illness. He viewed health and sickness as part of a continuum, using a play on words by calling it "health-ease" versus "dis-ease." It is not just health that moves on a continuum. Continuum means that within humans, there is a broad range of experiences. Continuum means that everybody is included.

As you will learn in detail in **Chapter 9** in the section on **Normal Distribution and the Bell Curve**, medicine these days tends to treat by the principle of what is called "evidence-based medicine." It usually means to treat with what works for the majority, unfortunately often leaving out considerable groups of people. To take full advantage of this book, the idea is to minimize categorization of "conditions" but follow as closely as possible your experience and underlying physiology. These are the areas where we have the most leverage to change most efficiently and effectively. We develop an understanding of what makes us tick and use it to our advantage at helping us live through cancer.

I'm not here to categorize your experience but to give you a chance to place yourself on the continuum of human existence and experience, understand your inner workings, and help you optimize your inner resources as you fight the tough battle with cancer.

WE ARE AS SIMPLE AS WE ARE COMPLEX

When we talk about continuum, we also need to discuss simplicity versus complexity, which as a concept moves on a continuum. Some things are simple, some things are complex. You will see me struggle throughout the book with when to apply simplicity and when to advocate complexity. Sometimes you will hear me emphasize simplicity, sometimes I will point out complexity. Sometimes I will reduce the complexity of our bodies to some simple principles as a guide to get through the horror of cancer, not out of disrespect for the miracle we are but for the practical necessity of survival while we are sick. Sometimes I will admonish you not to be too simplistic and instead respect the complexity of your situation. You will see me go back and forth between general ideas about humankind and cancer-specific examples because I believe that being a person with cancer is simply a subset of being a person. I will move around with you on the continuum of existence to match wherever you are at any given time.

Modern science is very complex and detailed. Even with many years of training and experience under my belt, I sometimes struggle to grasp the content of scientific literature. So I fully understand that it's even harder for laypeople to make sense of it. Add the distress of cancer, and it becomes almost impossible to decipher relevant content from the flood of highly complex information. I will only touch on the depth of some scientific complexity like brain research but will then synthesize the current knowledge into a consumer relevant denominator and translate it into practical action.

It is not just Cartesian dualism that can be a stumbling block to well-being for cancer patients. The complexity of medical knowledge can lead you into a suffocating jungle of choices. You are confronted with well-meaning advice ranging from juice fasts to complex targeted therapies and everything in between. I know you want to "get it right" because not "getting it right" might mean death, even if in reality this is often not true. How to pick and what to pick when is daunting. After all, despite all the advances in medicine, as we've seen science is not without errors.

The fact that we are complex—and that we do not understand all the underlying mechanics of human existence—makes it tempting to simplify complex processes. That is not per se wrong as long as we know that we are simplifying. It is when simplification becomes dogma that things can get dicey. Humans also attribute forces other than laws of chemistry and electronics to our existence. Abstraction is a very essential part of being a human. I doubt that a dog or cat think "I am worried that my cancer is going to kill me." It is an innately human thought; it is an abstract thought with a basis in a real-life event, namely some cells not following the rules of a coordinated effort of the body.

Every time you think an abstract thought, something very concrete and real happens inside your body. Sometimes the thought has a basis in reality; sometimes it is just a thought. It takes a series of complex chemical and electronic processes to make that thought happen. The thought itself is at least a nuisance, but the trickledown effect into other parts of the body complicates things further. Thinking repetitiously that you will die from cancer (even if you do not) can tense your muscles or cause a pit in your stomach. Understanding some of the underlying mechanics will give you more leverage to facilitate desired change.

A WORD ON INTEGRATION

So far in this book, we have encountered a discussion on "mind" and a discussion on "neuroplasticity." You also need to be comfortable with the word "integration." It is a word you will encounter a lot. Google's definition of the word *integration* as "the action and process of integration" is not very enlightening. What does integration really mean, and does the need for integration apply to you?

Google also offers definitions for "integration" in the area of psychology, "the coordination of processes in the nervous system, including diverse sensory information and motor impulses" and psychoanalysis, "the process by which a well-balanced psyche becomes whole as the developing ego organizes the id, and the state that results or that treatment seeks to create or restore by countering the fragmenting effect of defense mechanisms." The psychology definition, "The coordination of processes in the nervous system, including diverse sensory information and motor impulses" is ultimately what I do for a living. I might want to have a little chat with the Google employee who programmed the psychoanalysis definition into the system about whether they have the faintest idea what "the developing ego organizes the id" means.

"Integration" has also become the basis for a mushrooming industry with the sole purpose of making money rather than improving quality, and it is not always immediately apparent what you might gain from "integration." My favorite is "work-life integration." It is corporate lingo for working 24/7 in the service of your employer. Be mindful about what you are integrating. If you are setting out to "integrate," try to define first what you want to integrate. Be savvy in separating slogans from serious enterprise in the offerings available.

I spend some of my working time at a Center for Integrative Medicine (I always tease people when they erroneously call it the Center for "Integrated" Medicine. I wish medical treatment would be "integrated" rather than just in the process of "integrating" with the goal of "integration" in some distant future). Integrative means in the process of integrating with the outcome of being "integrated" as the end product. What exactly are we even integrating? East and West, conventional with complementary medicine, body and mind, psychiatry with neurology, primary care with specialty care?

As a cancer patient, you will find many offerings for "Integrative Oncology." Ask yourself and the person who offers the service what exactly they are planning to integrate? Are they going to facilitate the process of communication with your conventional oncologist? Are they going to educate you about treatments other than chemotherapy, radiation, and surgery? Are they going to help make decisions about a combination of treatments?

I appreciate the efforts of an ever-growing group of people to make us "whole" and "integrated" again. The irony is not lost on me, however, that when it comes to integrating body and mind, and psychiatry and neuroscience, that we have to painstakingly reverse a process that started in a philosopher's head but transformed and permeated into a society-dominating dogma in general. Yes, I am talking about Cartesian dualism.

When I talk about "integration," I briefly want to touch on a particular expertise I have. Many people seek me out specifically because they do not want to use medication to alter their mood or thinking. The reasons are varied. Some want to optimize their physiology naturally. A common argument I also hear is that patients do not want to add more medication to the already at times grueling cancer treatment regimen which, while eliminating cancer cells, also has an impact on healthy cells. Most often I wholeheartedly support the request, particularly since it is my particular skill to help people change without the use of medication. However, there is one area where I sometimes deviate from this concept, which is sleep. I am going to refer back to Mr. Baldwin to help us in the spiral process of going from unconscious incompetence to conscious incompetence and hopefully beyond.

As we have seen, getting a cancer diagnosis automatically constitutes distress. This in turn will alter your emotional and cognitive experience as you saw in Figure 5 (internalized yet?). Many of you know what it feels like to lie awake at night and think thoughts you'd rather not think. Unfortunately these thoughts impact your emotions and the nervous system. Now you can probably see why Mr. Baldwin is running (mental) circles at night. Whatever it takes to interrupt running circles, I will do. Sledgehammer aside. If you are one of those people affected by insomnia, you can go straight to section **Sleep Disturbance** in **Chapter 11** and **Chapter 13**. It might give you some relief.

Am I getting any closer to convincing you that it is beneficial to think of humans as a heap of cells, especially when it comes to your cancer? A reasonably designed and coordinated heap of cells but just a heap of cells after all (with plenty of kinks and the miracle of being able to cohabitate). I hope I have also started to persuade you that misinterpretations and misunderstandings of the function of these cells have led to misconceptions of human functioning, like the belief that body and mind are separate. I hope I have convinced you that you have to move thoughtfully in the ocean of knowledge if you want the best care as a cancer patient.

Our frame of reference is not always based in reality. Our thinking is heavily biased to suit ourselves. As a result, there is unnecessary suffering. And I hope I have also convinced you that integration of all our cells into one organic creature is advantageous. I have also argued that having a better understanding of your heap of cells will allow you to experience more well-being while going through the hell of cancer. That expansion of knowledge is related to growth.

Are you ready to take the role of your brain-maintenance engineer? How am I going to expand your knowledge of your own personal heap of cells? I will provide you with information, and I will also help you store the information and consolidate it in your brain. I mentioned in **The Preface** that the book is divided into a first part that addresses general principles of human physiology, anatomy, and biology, which is followed by parts devoted to cancer-specific issues. I had encouraged you to jump back and forth between the introductory chapters and the cancer-specific chapters that are most relevant to you. It will help with consolidation of knowledge and also facilitate to effectively act on your expanding insights.

If we understand the machine, the heap of cells that I will sometimes lovingly call "You" or "I," we are better equipped to maintain it and fix it when it is broken. What differentiates us from a car is the complexity of our mechanics. But the cells we are made of follow laws of chemistry and electricity that in essence are not different from the makings of a computer or a rat. After all, as we have seen, mind is "a relational and embodied process that regulates the flow of energy and information." I like this definition not just for the mind but for the rest of the body. Let's have your energy and information flow also.

INTERESTED IN CHANGE, ANYBODY?

I assume you are reading this book because you would like to change something. Whatever it is, your thoughts about cancer, your relationship with others, your headaches or sleepless nights. Change can happen naturally, or we can choose it, or it is thrust upon us. Some of this change comes as natural growth with the course of life maturation, but growth through cancer is usually in the "thrust upon us" category. Having cancer thrust upon them, patients often feel deprived of natural maturation that comes with aging. If we believe research, aging makes us more conscientious, kinder, calmer, confident, and caring (Caspi et al., 2005). I frequently hear people describe a sense of urgency for insight and growth as they fear their lifespan might be shortened. They wish to make up for the complacency they feel they may have had about their health. They develop a heightened sense of their mortality and want to pack a lifetime into the brief period they think they have left. This is particularly true for younger patients, as they have not gone through natural life cycles yet.

I have heard of people changing overnight, but in general I do believe that growth is gradual. Insight and enlightenment can be immediate and feel so illuminating and exhilarating that we are ready to change ourselves and the world overnight. The implementation into daily life, however, seems to be a more gradual process. I have always been grateful to people who have added insight and opportunity for change to my own life, and I happily want to do the same for you. My aim in this book is to help facilitate gradual change but also "expansion at a faster speed." Developing awareness that feels like maturation and allows for change.

Buddhist teacher Sharon Salzberg in her book, *Real Happiness*, describes it beautifully. While I am not happy with the title (real happiness as supposed to fake happiness?), her book on meditation is a good start for people who want to go down that road. She writes that "life holds moments when our perspective dramatically shifts, when our assumptions are deeply challenged." She suggests that change happens when either "a flash of inspiration or pain kick open that door."

"In our distress, we suddenly feel an urgent need to look more deeply for understanding and abiding sense of well-being." Ultimately there seems to be something mysterious about changing that we cannot evoke simply by pressing a button.

WHAT MAKES US CHANGE?

What do you do if you don't have the luxury of gradual, natural maturation because cancer has thrust you into life's abyss? I am afraid that crisis and adversity are bigger motivators than day-to-day life. Many of my patients, as soon as they get sick, become determined to eat healthy, exercise, meditate, and never again be mean to their children. Once the immediate threat of the illness has receded, old habits resurface. There seems to be a pull to revert to what is most familiar and habituated, or as a friend of mine pointed out, to sit in your shit is by no means pleasant, but it is at least warm and familiar. William James, one of my heroes who many consider the father of modern American psychology, already proclaimed in the 1890's that humans are creatures of habit. But that does not automatically mean we are doomed as he also contemplated how to use habituation to induce positive change. But let's start with the one I commonly see.

Suffering

Suffering as stimulator. Illness as emotional incubator. A ticket to personal liberation. I hear it from cancer patients all the time, "I wish I didn't have to get cancer to change my ways." Or to use a quote by James Lowell, "One thorn of experience is worth a whole wilderness of warning." The world is full of examples. Some of you might know the work of Oliver Sacks, who wrote many wonderful books about the brain and human experience. He himself was diagnosed with melanoma many years ago. At the time, he was told that he had a 2 percent chance of the cancer recurring. That means only two in 100 people in his situation would get sick again. I would happily settle for those odds if I got cancer. That also means ninety-eight of 100 people will be cured. Despite the good odds, he took his illness as an opportunity to live with what he called "relevance." For him personally, it meant starting to become very prolific with his writing. He devoted more and more time to writing.

His story reminds me of another writer who had a day job in Los Angeles and limited his writing to early morning hours before his nine to five job. At forty-one John Lescroart developed meningitis and was in a coma for eleven days. Upon waking up, he decided to quit his day job and become a full-time writer. He is now seventy-four, lives in the quaint, peaceful town of Davis in California, and has written almost thirty thrillers.

My patient Manuel experienced relevance differently altogether. He had a rare form of cancer that made his life span fairly unpredictable. When asked what the difference was between living one year versus ten years, he paused.

"If I had known for sure I would live ten more years, I would not have developed the ability to say 'no.' Assuming that I will live only one, I allow myself to say 'no' more often." Does only the face of illness and death make us change and allow us to say "no?"

But it is not just suffering that makes us grow. It is the fear of suffering that makes us *not* grow. I once overheard a workshop leader at Esalen, a personal growth retreat on the California coast, declare that people do not want to change because change is painful. Anyone who has ever wanted to stop smoking, eat healthier, or start to exercise knows how difficult it can be despite our best intentions. There seems to be an overruling human drive NOT to make changes and feel guilty about it instead. As usual it is important to acknowledge our individual differences and not judge our propensity to, at times, not want to change. We need to take seriously the molasses we can get stuck in and understand how it is motivated. I hope this book inspires you to change not just through suffering *and* to find inspiration that change itself does not constitute suffering.

Curiosity

Despite my clinical experience that suffering is an impetus to grow, I still believe that growth is possible from a place other than adversity and catastrophe alone. Many humans seem to go through some transformation during their lifetime. And I don't believe that the vast ocean of options to facilitate growth is just commercially driven. People often yearn for something other than what is. The various strands of the vast web of the self-growth industry often seem to intersect with similar recommendations. And personal paths of self-exploration often share similarities. A friend's discovery of the Vietnamese Buddhist master teacher Thich Nhat Hanh's *The Miracle of Mindfulness* made me immediately remember that Thich Nhat Hanh's book had left me with an important epiphany when I read it many years ago. I enjoyed that we encountered the same book as meaningful on our journey of growth. This book aids the intention and aspiration of growth. I hope that the other books I mention throughout this book become a meaningful reading list for you. Even though not necessarily intended that way originally, the shared experience through books, even when read at different times for different reasons, still creates a sense of community and belonging.

Need for Control, Anybody?

Looking at it from a different perspective, we could also call it "what makes us succeed" rather than grow.

Cancer patients have very common and shared experiences that they would like to experience differently. We can call it growth, success, change—whatever words suit you. The basic idea is to understand how, when you experience unpleasant state "x," you can shift to a pleasant state "y" efficiently, smoothly, and pleasantly. Can we include some factors and guidelines into our lives that ease the hardship?

We have known for a long time that it is not just suffering itself that is the challenge but suffering we feel we cannot control. Research on what is known as learned helplessness has shown that when people feel like they have no control over what happens, they tend simply to give up and accept their fate. This observation was based on a by now-famous experiment by Marty Seligman on dogs. Dogs that were given the option to end a five-second lasting shock early by pressing a panel were more proactive in escaping from future unpleasant situations than dogs that were conditioned to endure the shock helplessly. The dogs that had been conditioned to an inescapable situation before became a whimpering mess, enduring—rather than trying to escape from—their predicament (Seligman & Maier, 1967). Without wanting to compare us magnificent creatures to (also magnificent) dogs, the discovery also holds true for humans. The sense of loss of control is a fundamental aspect for cancer patients, which can lead to hopelessness and despair. When we come from lives with a reasonable sense of control, a cancer diagnosis can propel us into a whirlwind of not having a sense of control. Eureka! My clinical observation had some foundation in someone's research.

Perseverance

Another aspect of how to succeed in making change is described in Angela Duckworth's *Grit*. The author makes a case that to succeed a combination of perseverance and passion are helpful. This is important for cancer patients. Cancer can easily evoke a desire to give up. Connecting to a sense of loss of control can be the basis to wanting to give up. I don't want to be too much of a cheerleader for positive psychology, but I believe that some components from positive psychology are helpful and **Chapter 7** devotes a section to it.

If you know that perseverance is important, you might imagine using positive thinking in that particular moment. Don't think of chemotherapy or radiation as something that goes on for months or years. Think of it as something that goes on for one minute at a time. Perseverance in the sense of, "I am going to endure this for one more minute and then another one while I focus my attention on my knitting or my coloring book or a hilarious movie featuring Melissa McCarthy." While perseverance is worth aspiring to while you are sick, passion is a lot to ask for. But maybe your condition still allows you to contemplate an opportunity you always wanted to seize, a dream you never had a chance to at least ponder.

Practice

As Edgar Degas is said to have said, "Only when he no longer knows what he is doing does the painter do good things." This quote points out that practice is part of getting to unconscious competence (to refer back to my earlier remarks about learning that were illustrated by Figure 1).

Many people at this point have heard about the 10,000-hour rule, the number of hours it takes to become proficient at something. The number was based on studies by K. Anders Ericsson in the 1990's, and his work was popularized by Malcom Gladwell's book *Outliers*. The basic idea is that you have to practice to get good at something. It makes a lot of sense of course, and in part I base my encouragement to change gradually on it. I recommend promoting and consolidating change by practice. This is part of the reason why I often bombard you with exercises. Practice, practice, practice. Remember from Figure 1 that the progression in learning is ascending from unconscious incompetence to conscious incompetence before you advance via conscious competence to unconscious competence. It takes many, many hours that competence in a particular area feels like second nature.

There has been opposition to this idea, too, since studies have also demonstrated that some people can get proficient with fewer hours and others who practice for even more hours don't. I don't consider this a valid argument to reject the proverb in German that states that "practice creates masters" (which I much prefer to "practice makes *perfect*"), particularly thinking about a bell curve (more details in **Chapter 9** in the section on **Normal Distribution and the Bell Curve**). I suspect the 10,000-hour rule applies to the majority of people, but that does not preclude some people getting good at something faster, or some people not getting good at something despite practicing a lot.

I hope I don't hear you say, "I don't have 10,000 hours. I am too busy with cancer." In order to benefit from what you are reading and the exercises here, you don't have to become a master violinist. I have referred to learning a language before. Starting with small pieces and gradually expanding on it will give you much satisfaction. Practice is just one piece of the puzzle.

Here and Now

The point is that both growth and change are gradual and happen most effectively with awareness in the moment. It is important to give yourself short breaks, even if it is just moments at a time. I observe that many people, not just sick ones, live in the notion that we must grind away at life now, and later we'll get some respite on a vacation far away—the week in Hawaii to recover from the Silicon Valley rat race or whatever your circumstances might be. This "on and off "mode is not really conducive to health. It is also not compatible with the anatomy and physiology of our bodies. We need to be able to sustain some level of continuity with respect to well-being. Going away to recover defeats the purpose. We will also look at how to consolidate change and growth. Practice and patience to become who we want to be.

A WORD ON THERAPIES AND HOW TO GET HELP

Growth and change are the words I want you to keep in mind if you seek help managing your feelings about cancer. I have urged you not to look at yourself as mentally ill. The same way it helps to understand what makes us grow and what prevents growth, we need to understand what is therapeutic.

Americans spend billions of dollars every year in the self-improvement market in the pursuit of happiness (LaRosa, 2013). With that much money spent, I would expect us all to be enlightened geniuses by now. As a cancer patient, you will be bombarded with suggestions about what you *should* do. While juice fasts, elimination of refined sugar, meditation, positive thinking, and spiritual practice can have a valid place in cancer care, I witness patients getting lost in the choices. Instead of doing things to improve their health, the multitude of choices adds stress.

I am often confronted with the question, "Are you doing CBT" (cognitive behavioral therapy), or by the clinical note, "patient referred for CBT"

"What is it exactly you are doing?"

"Ah! Mh!" are not answers that instill confidence in my future clients. I do, however, struggle with the answer. I am often tempted to answer that my expertise is "well-being." That, however, is not really doing the question justice. I often don't know how to respond since I do not want to limit my treatment to one modality. My answer often is that of course I work with "cognition" and "behavior," which is true but still doesn't address the question.

I find the confines of therapeutic modalities very limiting. Most available interventions and therapies aim at well-being or at least claim to do so. If the word "salutogenesis" that I already introduced you to weren't so exotic, I would probably call myself a salutogenesist.

The basic idea is that you fit the technique to the person, not the person to the technique. I have emphasized the uniqueness of each person on the continuum of existence. Finding help means finding a doctor and healthcare team who can recognize that and have options for change.

The same way I want you to master the laws of thought and emotion to lighten your life the way a martial arts master integrates the laws of gravity and leverage to effortlessly flatten an opponent, competent "salutogenesis" providers need to be able to effortlessly and competently suspend themselves and their own needs to be able to grasp your individuality and your individual needs to be able to help you. This is not always easy to find as providers, particularly at the beginning of their career, set out with a one-size-fits-all approach, and the nuances necessary to adapt to every individual take time and experience. Don't be shy about shopping around to separate the wheat from the chaff.

While this is human and reflects the helper's expansion and professional growth, it also represents the provider's inability to live with inexperience. The same way patients struggle with uncertainty, so do providers. They want to feel competent and prefer to have techniques they feel comfortable with rather than recognize that some of these techniques might not fit you. The best way to succeed is to be literally in the moment, very quickly assess what is in the moment and make an adjustment to optimize outcome. Humbly working on improving your techniques.

The undertaking to find the most effective help requires identifying your problems and your goals first. Are you someone who is mostly bothered by thought intrusions that keep you up at night? Are you someone who bursts into tears at the drop of a hat? Or do you notice mysterious aches and pains all over your body that someone told you are "psychological" or "psychosomatic?" Do you prefer to cathartically express your thoughts and emotions or to take action on your insights?

Always remember that we treat all cells equally. Identify and define what you experience, preferably without giving it a diagnostic label and ask whoever you are seeking help from the following questions.

"I have noticed x, y, and z. Can you help me with this? How would you help me? What is involved? How long will it take and how much will it cost?"

Don't assume that an education from a prestigious school is the ticket to success. The health market outside of conventional medicine is huge.

Also, follow your gut and recommendations from trusted friends. Don't think of yourself as someone with a mental problem. Think of yourself as a heap of cells. A heap of cells in distress.

I witnessed an interaction between a physician and a patient that piqued my interest. When the doctor asked if the patient thought she was depressed, the patient answered, "I have cancer." Your heap of cells has challenges because part of the heap are cancer cells, not because you are mentally disturbed. The most simple rule of all: If the person you seek help from uses the word "should" more than five times during the first visit, I recommend not going back. The very concept of "should" impedes growth. Remember the quote from the patient earlier who promised herself to never use the word "should" again.

As a cancer patient, you will often find yourself confronted with your own beliefs. That process can be quite surprising and often upsetting. But the information unearthed in the process can also be illuminating, even liberating. There is a soft spot where growth happens. Anybody who has ever learned to drive a stick shift car will understand. There is this magic spot when you gently let go of the clutch while gently pressing the accelerator and the car moves. Human growth is similar. And when the car stalls, you can always turn it back on.

PART II

GENERAL CONCEPTS

In order to make use of this book, you'll need to be familiar with some basic concepts from psychology, anatomy, physiology, and neuroscience. I'm going to present some core concepts in reasonable depth but always with references for literature that allows for deepening understanding or particular interests.

The first step is to recall Figure 5. It is a reminder how important thoughts, emotions, and body sensations are for us humans. In discussing questions of anatomy and physiology, it will be more important to understand the physiology of those components than how exactly a cell in the liver or the kidney works. The red arrows remind you that thoughts, emotions, and physical sensations are also closely interrelated. You don't have to concentrate yet on what the car represents, but we will talk about it in detail in **Chapter 3**.

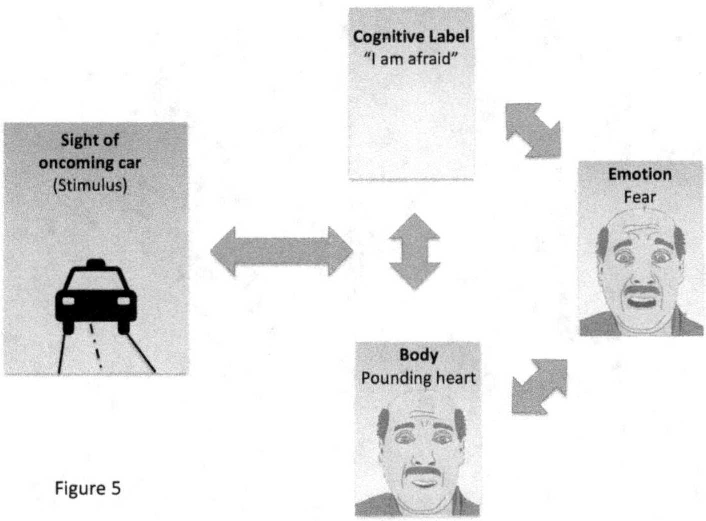

Figure 5

While I was writing the book's different sections on body, emotion, and thinking, I felt increasingly conflicted about the lack of true separateness of these three entities. I wanted to stay within the theoretical framework but also wanted to be true to the individual nuances of these concepts and considerable overlap in the reality of life. They are all closely interrelated and overlappingly mixed. Thought affects emotion, and emotion affects thought. Emotions and thoughts affect body, and body affects emotion and thought. We'll look at this bi-directionality through some amusing and illuminating studies.

CHAPTER 2.

Thought-Body-Emotion: A Love-Jealousy Triangle

While you are reading about the connection of thought, emotion, and the "rest of the body," I want you to be aware that these entities at times fiercely fight and compete for attention and other times synergistically collaborate. I encourage you to learn the rules of these systems, so you can optimize their collaboration rather than be weighed down by the fights. No different from a marriage. Know, too, that they are in constant communication.

BODY AND EMOTIONS ARE TWINS CONJOINED AT THE HIP

I want you to observe how you feel and what you think about when you slouch vs. when you sit upright. Can you try both positions and see? Take your time while also focusing on your breathing in one position before you change to the other. I encountered a study that reported that students who are instructed to do their homework in a slouching position are more likely to be depressed after a few weeks than students instructed to do their homework in an upright posture (Veenstra et al., 2016). And it works in the opposite direction as well. People with depression improved their affect, fatigue, and verbal expression by focusing on being in an upright position (Wilkes et al., 2017). Body and emotions, and body and mood (a sibling to emotions as you will learn in the chapter on emotions) are closely related! And it goes both ways, thus my use of the word bidirectional.

How you sit affects your emotions and your mood, and your emotions and your mood affect how you sit. Most people are not surprised that their mood might affect their body posture, literally "being down." When presented with the data of the study, they chuckle, however, at the thought that their body posture might affect their mood. But it has important implications. Straighten up, everybody! It takes little effort to occasionally straighten up. It is a physiological freebee. As a cancer patient, you have no time or energy to spare. I encourage you to integrate tools that are easy and effective. Like sitting upright if it feels energizing and your illness allows. Even when you are confined largely to the bed or couch, you can try to sit upright and not slouch.

As the study on the students is an illustration of how your body impacts your emotions, now I want to give you an example of how your emotions impact your body beyond just your posture.

Studies show that happy people more easily fight off a common cold (Cohen et al., 2003). The fact that our emotional states and mood are related to health is stressful to cancer patients as they often struggle with questions of how they might have caused their cancer because they were presumably not happy enough or relaxed enough or aware enough. I don't want to add distress with this finding but simply make you aware of how closely emotions and body interact and hopefully motivate you to pay attention. At no point do I ever want anyone to walk away with the idea that your emotional state *causes* cancer as I mentioned very early in the book when mentioning distress and health. This kind of thinking is too simplistic and causes much suffering. Development of cancer is intricately complex. The important distinction here is that, yes, distress, mood, emotions, and even your body position affect your health, but cancer is not your fault, and you did not *cause* it. In the chapter on emotions, we will go deeper and differentiate mood from feelings and emotion, but for now we can throw them in one bucket as entities that communicate with the body and vice versa.

It takes time to untangle the misconceptions about the body's connections. Learning how emotions and body are connected took me quite a while. I remember vividly being introduced to the idea that emotions were "stored in the body" while spending time at Esalen Institute. Trained scientist that I am, my mind desperately tried to figure out how that was possible. Looking back I chuckle.

Feeling emotions while physically touched during a massage made it seem plausible that "emotions are stored in the body." Could the emotion have somehow gotten into the DNA of a muscle cell? Could the cell contain chemicals that correlated with emotions? I was thinking hard. Now it seems so obvious to me that the emotion is stored in the brain (more differentiated details about that in **Chapter 5** on **Emotions**), and similar to the example of the slouching students, there is a physical correlate in our muscles when we experience an emotion. I am not sure why it took me ten years to understand that, but it did.

Remembering my own bewilderment, I have a lot of compassion for patients who stare at me blankly when I talk about the bidirectional connection between emotion and body. I won't tell them that emotions are stored in the body, but I might borrow words from the brilliant title of Bessel van der Kolk's book, *The Body Keeps the Score*. The title of another book, *Your Body Believes Every Word You Say*, sums it up more humorously.

The cells in our body are very interrelated. Cells in the brain that create an emotion are closely connected to muscles in the periphery through nerves. Maybe you can relate to the experience of being a lousy passenger. I definitely am. I had to teach myself not to shriek when my husband drove, but I still clasped the door handle rigidly, and my foot hit an imaginary brake. Anticipatory fear and muscle tension are closely related! The underlying need of course is to control. It feels much better to be the one who has control over not crashing into the wall than surrendering your destiny in the passenger seat.

BODY AND THOUGHTS ARE TWINS CONJOINED AT THE HIP

Most people do not realize how closely their thoughts are linked to their body. Catherine, whom you met on the first pages of this book, illustrated it firsthand. Her body was driven by the sentence, "I can do this, no matter what." "This" in her life referred to pretty much anything. Her body was running around like a lunatic in order to prove it. "I can do this, no matter what." Her body complied until she got sick. But all of a sudden, her sick body could not keep up with her mental expectation. She was not a happy camper.

Over time she learned to follow her husband's signal to slow down whenever he made a specific hand motion. She laughingly stated that she needed an external brake keeper, otherwise her body would keep trying to execute on her thought that she "could do it, no matter what." Because some of these entities are so intertwined, it can be helpful to separate them. More awareness helps with change. Catherine had to be aware of her underlying thought in order to avoid automatically having her body execute on it.

Many studies show that our thoughts and expectations influence our bodies. Ellen Langer, the first woman to get tenure in the department of psychology at Harvard University, has set up many experiments to demonstrate the connection. In an experiment in the 1980's, she placed elderly gentleman from a nursing home in surroundings that resembled their life twenty years earlier. They were instructed not to just reminisce about their earlier life but also to act like the person they were twenty years earlier.

Within a week, the gentlemen in the group acting as if they were twenty years younger showed several advantages over the control group, who went about their business as usual. They were physically more flexible, sat taller, and most improbable, their eyesight improved (Langer, 2009). In an article in the *New York Times* in 2014, Langer told the reporter that the "men had put their mind in an earlier time, and their bodies went along for the ride" (Grierson, *New York Times*, October 22, 2014).

In another study, she informed hotel chambermaids who self-reported that they didn't get much exercise in a typical week that cleaning rooms constitutes exercise. Nothing other than their expectations were shifted, and the ladies lost weight compared to their fellow workers who had not been given the information (Crum & Langer, 2007).

Unfortunately it's not just positive messages that sink in. This is particularly important for cancer patients. In another study, Langer found that breast cancer patients who describe themselves as "in remission" had more pain than women who considered themselves "cured." Notably the patients were not different with respect to their cancer. She recommends using language mindfully, a suggestion I wholeheartedly endorse. In her vocabulary, the words "victim" and "cancer" don't go in the same sentence.

I vividly remember a patient named Berta, who tearfully reported on her first visit that she was "terminal." Inquiring what that meant, she could not illuminate. Her oncologist, whom she pressed for his definition of "terminal" on her next visit, wavered. He simply had meant to express that he could not cure Berta and that he could not give her a timeline on how long she was going to live.

My heart went out to Berta, as the word "terminal" to both of us implied that Berta was "dying soon." That meaning of "terminal" is very different from what her oncologist had meant to say. I still see her occasionally, and we both laugh when we remember the ominous word "terminal" that like the "Dark Lord" in Harry Potter better remains unspoken, unless of course it is an assessable reality.

Even well-meant mindsets (I use the word with the broad meaning of "belief" rather than the more defined meaning popularized by the social psychologist Carol Dweck) get in the way of your well-being. Yolanda had gone through a harrowing experience with cancer twice, leaving her with considerable lymphedema in her right arm, making her life as a software engineer challenging. She, however, also felt deep gratitude towards the people who had helped her through the process.

After she came out at the end of her own dark tunnel of illness, she was determined to help others. Whenever there was an opportunity to guide other people through the process of cancer, she would volunteer. She had a strong belief that "I need to pay back the cancer community." While she certainly meant well, she didn't realize how being exposed to the world of cancer was distressful to her as it was a constant reminder of what she had gone through and also instilled fears about a cancer recurrence in the future.

Her experience made it emotionally difficult to discern other peoples' stories from her own. Once she could change her mindset from "I have to help people with cancer" to "I want to help," she felt better as she could shift her attention towards helping people with ailments other than cancer without paying the price of being fearful about her own situation.

EMOTIONS AND THOUGHTS ARE TWINS CONJOINED AT THE HIP

Just as body and thought and body and emotions are conjoined twins, emotions and thoughts are as well. The easiest way to demonstrate this connection is with an exercise. Just take a moment to assess whether or not you feel well. Do you have pleasant or unpleasant thoughts? Is your body relaxed or restless? Then take a moment to remember a situation when someone crossed you or someone treated you unfairly. Maybe you were laid off or passed over for a promotion. Maybe your partner filed for divorce and you still hurt. How does thinking about the event change your emotions? Do you notice anger welling up? Not everybody has a strong reaction, but simply notice if you have a change in emotion based on the thoughts and memories.

You can also do the exercise imagining a pleasant scene. Do your emotions shift back to something more pleasant? In my clinical experience, it is much easier to connect to negative emotions than to positive emotions by thinking something negative or positive respectively. And I get support from science for my observation. Science calls this phenomenon negativity bias, and the psychologist Rick Hanson is known for his expression that "in effect the brain is like Velcro for negative experiences but Teflon for positive ones" (Hanson & Mendius, 2009). Negative experiences easily get stuck in our thinking, and scientist have examined the amount of positive feedback necessary to outweigh the negative—the so-called positivity ratio. There has been considerable debate in scientific circles around the notion what that exact ratio might be (Fredrickson & Losada, 2005, Friedman & Brown, 2018) but no debate about negativity bias itself.

Winnifred Gallagher, whom you already met in the section on **Salutogenesis** in **Chapter 1**, supports my clinical observation with research. She presents several examples from research illustrating our negativity bias. You reportedly listen longer to complaints about yourself than compliments, and you're more likely to see an angry face in the crowd of happy people than a happy face in a crowd of angry people. These are two examples that she uses to further speculate that from an evolutionary perspective attending to negative thoughts and emotions might promote survival.

Even if that were true, I think it is time that we help evolution catch up to our current intellectual abilities. I often challenge my patients when they try to convince me that focusing on every ache and pain and getting monthly MRIs will keep them safe. While I feel compassion for the motive driving their desire, I more often witness distress from this coping style than a feeling of safety. To promote health, we are confronted with the challenge to create positivity and optimism despite an evolutionarily sound negativity bias. Oh boy, who says life is easy? Add cancer, and the task can feel daunting. Since negativity bias is heavily driven by thought, **Chapter 4** on **Thinking** will provide several sections with practices to help counter this negativity bias.

ADVOCATING FOR PURITY

If everything in our body is so entwined, why my yearning for purity to isolate emotions, thoughts, and body sensations? Monitoring these components individually serves as an alert system that says, "hey, something is going on, pay attention." A whiff of sadness, some chest discomfort, a peculiar thought. "Pay attention, these are signals for potentially useful additional information."

These signals that serve as connectors to more information are particularly important as a lot of mental processing happens outside of our conscious awareness, as you are about to read in the section **Incognito** in **Chapter 3**. Paying attention to the individual components is a step that helps us change. Remember the analogy to dancing? We evolve from unconscious incompetence by developing awareness. Being aware of what happens inside us helps develop competence not just on the dance floor but on the cancer floor.

Throughout the remainder of the book, I will encourage you to distill your experience into components while acknowledging that the individual pieces are meshed in complex ways. Letters make words, and words make sentences, but even Shakespeare started with letters first. By no means does this reductionist approach mean I am not aware of the complexity of our existence. The simplification allows us easier access to our complexity. Emotions, thoughts, and physical sensations become building blocks of insight.

CHAPTER 3.

How We Process Events

In **Chapter 2** we focused on how closely thought, emotion, and physical experiences are bidirectionally connected to each other. In this chapter, we will focus on what happens to these building blocks of insight when something happens outside of you and you react to it. When I introduced you to Mr. Baldwin earlier, I called this exchange a constant back-and-forth between the external world and our internal world and compared it to playing a round of table tennis. Let's experience this exchange with a little exercise. If you can't retrieve Figure 5 from memory, here's a little reminder to assist you.

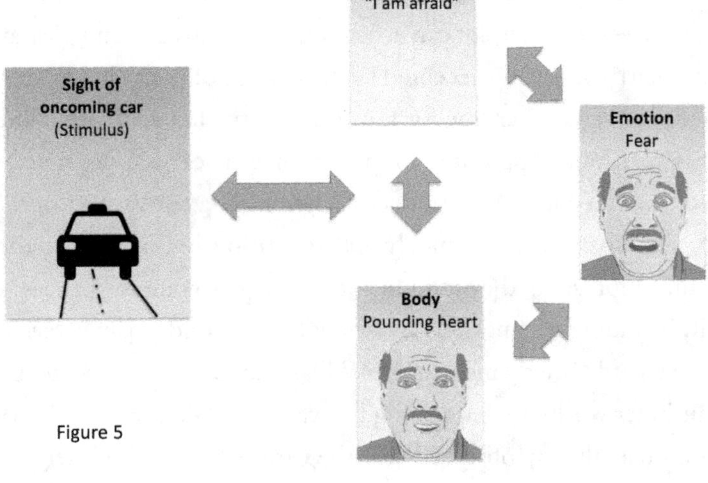

Figure 5

Take a moment to reflect on what you experience when a car cuts you off or you accidentally step in front of a car on the crosswalk. Slow down your breathing, so you can reflect on your thoughts, experience your feelings, and notice your body responses in this scenario. Are you someone whose heart will beat faster, feel scared, or be thinking about the car driving at you? Or will you be thinking about the fact that you are scared? This is an experience most of us have had in our lives. The image illustrates a framework of how humans respond to an external event with emotions, thoughts, and body responses. It depicts your reaction when a car drives at you or cuts you off. And as you know from experience, that can be quite stressful.

Always keep in mind that there are individual differences in our responses. Some people will curse like sailors when they get cut off, others will physically shake from fear while others will feel sad about the thoughtlessness or rudeness of other people. But the central point is that most of us will react. In case you were wondering why I started the book with an awareness exercise on thought, emotion, and body. Now you know why!

Scientists have argued whether emotion and physical response happen consecutively or concurrently, but for the purposes of this book and the exercises that were developed from it, the precise timing and physiology do not matter. What matters is that Mr. Baldwin represents the roadmap that is now your internal companion.

This framework of how we react to the external world does not just refer to negative stressors. An event can evoke something positive and pleasant, such as getting married, getting accepted to the college of your choice, or hearing that you have been cancer free for ten years! As the last sentence alludes, this concept is very much applicable to cancer since cancer is a negative event to most people. The concept presented in Figure 5 is a core aspect of this book and will accompany you intimately and repetitiously throughout the book. The picture represents the simplification of a very complex process of how our body, including its emotions and thoughts, responds to an external event.

I have already briefly mentioned William James who was quite insightful about our inner world not happening in a vacuum. As far back as the 19th century, James had already observed that the external world is closely linked to the internal world, but he had no means of proving it since, at the time, scientists could not measure nerve activation or biochemicals like the "stress hormone" cortisol. Like Semmelweis' ideas, James' were novel and not universally accepted at the time, but unlike Semmelweis, James enjoyed an illustrious academic career. When I discovered James' work, it felt as if all of a sudden several puzzle pieces of understanding fell into place. Patients also seem to be able to relate their own experience to James' concept, thus encouraging me further to use it as a tool to facilitate health and well-being. His ideas have evolved over time as scientists were able to take a closer look at what happens inside of us.

I hope my arguments have convinced you why Mr. Baldwin represents the roadmap that is now your internal companion. The relevant information can be boiled down to this: WHEN SHIT HITS THE FAN, THE MACHINE WE CALL "I" WILL REACT. YOUR HEAP OF CELLS WILL GO INTO SURVIVAL MODE. YOUR THOUGHTS, EMOTIONS, AND BODY MIGHT EVEN GO A LITTLE APESHIT.

A TRUCK JUST RAN ME OVER

When cancer is the "event," the metaphor might more aptly be to getting run over by a runaway truck! The "event" cancer has an impact on our body, our emotions, and our thinking. Every aspect of the "event" cancer can become a stressor that finds its way into our thinking, our emotion, and our body. I purposely use the words thought, body, and emotion to stay consistent with the picture presented in Figure 5. When I use the word "body," I always refer to the totality of a human being, to every piece and cell that we are made of, our heap of cells that I consistently keep referring to. We will talk about "stress" and "stressor" in more detail, but for now we're talking about an event than evokes something inside of us.

In this context, I want to remind you of the conversation about mind. I expect some of you to object to the information that emotions and thoughts are creations of the body. But remember that the many scientists debating with Dan Siegel about what mind was concluded that emotions and thought have to do with mind, and mind has to do with brain. And since the brain is part of the body, so must be emotions and thought. I hope Socrates would be proud of my deductive reasoning.

If you take naturally to this idea, you can ignore the next three paragraphs, but if you are like me and at first stumbled over the notion that emotions are brain based, read on. Simply replace the word "body" with a picture of yourself or another human being. When you read the word "body" in this book, it always refers to the totality of you, to the whole heap of cells.

I emphasize this point to try to avoid confusion as to the word "body" being used as contrast to a concept that many humans experience as "bodiless," such as "mind" or "spiritual." I want to hammer home the point that "mind" is "body" (or at least is closely related to body) to optimize your knowledge about how your heap of cells operates, not because I disregard thoughts about spirituality or abstraction of thought.

I notice that I am not the only one struggling to come up with a nomenclature that is distinctive. Lisa Feldman Barrett, a psychology professor at Northeastern University, in her book *How Emotions Are Made*, uses the word "body" to mean everything but the brain. When she refers to the entire body including the brain, she uses the term "anatomical body." While I understand her reasoning, her nomenclature suggests that the brain is separate from the body. In this book, the word "body" includes the totality of you, every cell, including brain cells. Ultimately the language about what constitutes "body" doesn't matter, as long as you know that emotions and thoughts are closely related to the brain.

EVERYBODY IS DIFFERENT

As I mentioned a moment ago in relation to getting cut off by a car, there are vast individual differences with respect to how people react to external events. When the stressor is cancer, some people will become more emotional, others oddly detached. Some will have sleepless nights, pounding hearts, and difficulty thinking. Some will become super rational; others find their thinking strangely altered. Did you have any of those responses when cancer knocked on your door? Or was your own response different? If you are long past your diagnosis, you can take a more recent example of an extremely stressful event to explore your response.

People can usually easily relate to the idea that our bodies, thoughts, and emotions react to events but might have different opinions with respect to the process of *how* that happens. The idea that everything stems from body (including the brain) is important as people often experience thoughts and emotions as abstractions rather than creations of their body. The reason for this is mostly cultural and historical, as I outlined earlier in our discussion of Cartesian dualism. The understanding is important, as people tend to have the misconception that emotions and thoughts are exclusively subject to will and control, which can add unnecessary distress. I want you to think of a human as one piece with different functions, such as a beating heart, a breathing lung, and a thought- and emotion-creating brain.

Did you stumble over the expression "emotion-creating brain?" Some people will reject the notion that emotions are mostly brain based, as many people tend to say their emotions come from the "heart." I say "mostly" as the reality as usual is more complex. I will elaborate in more detail in **Chapters 5 and 6** on **Emotion** and **Body** as we work our way into deeper understanding of our inner makings. It might sound strange, but what you will learn later on in the book is that we can identify some emotional states by observing heart rate variations. But before you reach for your wrist to feel your pulse, read closely that I did not say heart rate but heart rate variations.

If you burn with curiosity what that means, you can peek at **Chapter 6** in the section on **The Heart**. Part of experiencing emotions coming from the heart has to do with the close connection of the brain with nerves that connect the heart to the brain and vice versa. We discussed that muscles can contract when we have emotions and so can the heart. It probably won't surprise you to hear that the heart is in fact a muscle. The heart often does experience something when we experience an emotion because of its close connection to the brain. You could say the heart is usually along for the ride when the brain creates an emotion.

CHANGING FROM WITHIN

Okay, I think we've established *that* we react to external events. People, however, have a harder time with the idea that *how we relate to* and think about the external event can have as much of an impact on our emotions and our thinking and can evoke as much of a stressful body response as the event itself. In fact thoughts and emotions can get stuck in stressful loops in our body. No one knows this better than you!

Many people have negative thoughts that they recognize as futile, which they don't want to think but think anyway, and they are stressed that they cannot NOT think them. Even when there is no event but only event-induced thoughts, for example memories of an event, these memory-based thoughts can speed up our heart rate and evoke a similar fearful state as if the event were happening right then and there.

I work with patients who have a vivid recollection of the time and location when they were informed about their cancer diagnosis. Even months or years later they have physical sensations when they think about that time or walk or drive past the location where the verdict was handed down.

At the beginning of this chapter, I had you practice with the image of Mr. Baldwin what this stressful reaction feels like. The red arrows show the interconnectedness of emotion, thoughts, and body going circular, and as you may well know, we can easily end up in a vicious cycle of body, thought, and emotions all feeding on each other. This phenomenon is another core concept of this book, and unpacking it is the basis of many of the practical exercises you already have been and will be consistently asked to try throughout the book. This expands my earlier statement about the shit hitting the fan.

Whereas before I said, "WHEN SHIT HITS THE FAN, THE MACHINE WE CALL 'I' WILL REACT," now we might say, "WHEN SHIT HITS THE FAN, THE MACHINE WE CALL 'I' WILL REACT IN WAYS THAT MIGHT HAVE ONLY LITTLE TO DO WITH THE SHIT THAT HIT THE FAN."

The underlying idea in this proposal is not new by the way. Epictetus, a teacher of Stoic ethics in ancient Greece and former slave, put it more eloquently when formulating in his writings that "it is not the things themselves that disturb man, but their judgments about these things" (Encheiridion, 5).

I can already hear the critics bang down my door. Let me elaborate. I am not suggesting that events do not have an impact on us or that we should strive not to respond. A cancer diagnosis is indeed devastating—no question—*and* I urge you to explore your internal response to it as we carry inside of us information that can be beneficial to heal and feel well. Even when upon first examination we want to focus solely on the event "cancer."

Victor Frankl, an Austrian physician, author and Holocaust survivor, put it beautifully, "Between stimulus and response there is a space. In that space is our power to choose our response. In our response lies our growth and our freedom." Allow yourself to explore that space. You will not regret it.

Writer and filmmaker Ruth Whippman in her book, *America the Anxious*, asks us to acknowledge that misery can simply be in our response to external circumstances. She takes issue with Eckhart Tolle's (a spiritual teacher who many of you may know as the author of *The Power of Now*) writing that "the primary cause of unhappiness is never the situation but your thoughts about it" (Sounds as if Tolle has heard of Epictetus also). While I agree with her criticism of "the happiness gurus, who insist that the real problems in our lives are never discrimination or poverty, bad relationships, or unfair bosses…but our own failure to adopt whatever the latest Big Happiness-endorsed thinking style might be, think positive or practice mindfulness, to take personal responsibility or count our blessings," I take issue mostly with Tolle's use of the word "never." I would say that "the primary cause of unhappiness is *often* not the situation but your thoughts about it."

As usual it boils down to trying to find an equilibrium between acknowledging the circumstances and exploring your response to it—as long as this helps your health and does not become just a navel-gazing waste of time and energy.

I might sound as if I am splitting hairs, but the differentiation is very important from a clinical perspective. Cancer patients commonly experience considerable distress from how they think about their circumstances. The situation of having cancer is stressful enough. The thought that you might have caused the cancer can add as much distress as the cancer itself. The isolation that is sometimes caused by the illness also can be as stressful as the illness itself.

Many of you have heard about the association of stress and illness and often end up feeling stressed about the stress you feel as you mentally connect to cancer progression or recurrence or other stressful thoughts. My point is you could not control that you got cancer, but you can do a lot not to add distress now that you have it.

You don't want to have cancer to begin with, but once you have it, you don't want to be bombarded by internal thoughts that are stressful on top of the stress of cancer. To help minimize discomfort, it is very important to keep separate what happens to you from how you think about it. We often have little control over our circumstances, but we can gain some control over how we think and feel in reaction to them. That's the whole point here.

TAKE ADVANTAGE OF YOUR SURROUNDINGS

On the bright side, even as I advocate for exploring your reaction to the event in order to minimize distress rather than be riled by it, I am all for taking advantage of the fact that our surroundings can also have an impact on us in a positive way. I already suggested that you integrate straightening your body into your daily routine. Similarly, as a cancer patient, you might want to request a room with a view. Some of you might have heard of the "window effect." Reviewing records from patients who had their gallbladder removed, we see that the patients whose room had a window looking out on nature had a shorter postoperative hospital stay, gave less negative feedback, and took less pain medication than patients who were facing a brick wall (Ulrich, 1984).

I often suggest to my patients that if they want to improve their mood, they can simply let their eyes rest on a pleasant or soothing image, such as one of nature or animals (and straighten up of course while you stare). You don't have to do anything other than passively let looking at something lovely evoke a corresponding effect inside of you.

Let's take advantage when our surroundings having a positive impact on us while learning to internally modify the negative impact of our less-desirable surroundings. I hope you will hit the woods when you learn that newly diagnosed cancer patients who interacted with a natural outdoor environment for just two hours once a week improved their ability to pay attention (Cimprich & Ronis, 2003).

BALANCING THE EXTERNAL WITH THE INTERNAL WORLD

As we go forward, we will further explore the intimate interaction of external events with internal responses to these events and the external world and how our internal world can shape our experience of the external world. I want to turn to how our bodies do that and how and why it does not seem coordinated perfectly. Our heap of cells has a reflexive survival function as all animals do, but it does not appear to have flawlessly coordinated perfection when doing so, and I am going to discuss a few possible reasons. I believe a lot lies in evolution and the development of thinking and cognition, and those abilities not being coordinated well with older parts of the brain, particularly under duress. Cancer constitutes duress. Van der Kolk puts it bluntly, stating that "the rational brain is basically incompetent to talk the emotional brain out of its own reality." Amen.

If that idea seems alien, just take a moment and try to remember a time when you took a walk in the woods at nighttime or were walking home from the movies late at night. You might have heard sounds. You might have felt a sense of unease. Your heart might have beaten a little faster. There was nothing there to evoke the fear, but you felt it anyway. You internally generated something related to danger, maybe a memory from summer camp as a child or not realizing that you were imagining a mugger behind the next tree. A reptile would not have the added thought content leading to misinterpretation of its surroundings.

My personal theory here is that the evolution of cognition has not been perfectly coordinated (yet?) with our instinctual reptilian existence, which is millions of years older. We are still evolving as humans, and we still need to evolve further, so we won't mistake the shadow of a tree for a robber. Or decide that our cancer will rob our children of our existence, even if it does not or might not for years.

INCOGNITO

Part of the disconnect I just described might be related to how the brain stores information, the lack of conscious access to that information, and the interference of that information with our choices. There is ample evidence that every conscious experience we have is stored in our brains. In the 1950's Wilder Penfield, a renowned American neurosurgeon working in Canada was poking around in people's brains to treat their seizures (Dittrich, 2016). He had already successfully mapped the parts of the brain that were responsible for movement and sensation by gently touching an electrode systematically throughout specific parts of the brain when he came upon a wondrous phenomenon. As Penfield touched parts of the medial temporal lobes, people would describe whole scenes, situations, and interactions. It soon became apparent that memories were being resurrected.

Try to imagine that all our experiences are stored in the brain. The thought is mindboggling. When you consider it, it is not surprising that little of this stored information is accessible to our consciousness; if it were, we would be chronically overwhelmed. The information rests somewhere in the collective heap of brain cells.

Could it be that all this stored but not accessible information is active inside us without our being aware? And not just active but determining our behavior? One of my favorite books of all times, David Eagleman's *Incognito*, subtitled *The Secret Lives of the Brain*, says yes and presents good evidence to prove it.

Not "life" but "lives" his title states! Oh, boy!

I had similarly powerful Eureka moments reading Eagleman's book as I had with William James' thoughts on emotion and body. All of a sudden, some of my own and other people's strange behavior and thoughts made perfect sense. Some of Eagleman's examples are quite amusing. The brain constantly collects information, makes assessments, and adapts behavior. These complex processes happen completely outside of our awareness. Eagleman calls consciousness a "tiny stowaway on the transatlantic steamship, taking credit for the journey without acknowledging the massive engineering underfoot." What a poignant metaphor embedded in beautiful language!

I use a study in my own teaching to make his point. If you ask men to rank women on their attractiveness based on a photo, the assessment will depend on whether or not the women's pupils were dilated prior to taking the photo. Men were more attracted to women with dilated eyes. The brains of the men saw something that the men themselves were not aware of. Dilated eyes correlate with sexual arousal and readiness (Lick et al., 2016). Who knew! The feminist in me wonders if this was studied in gender reverse, but I suspect not.

I am not suggesting that people start dilating their pupils before their next date, but I want us all to start acknowledging that we are guided by brain activity outside our awareness. The brain does have a life of its own.

Another intriguing example is described in Malcolm Gladwell's *Blink*. Gladwell describes the training of chicken sexers (looking for an intriguing job anyone?). Apparently it is important to differentiate the sex of chicks after birth. And we learn that it is difficult to determine the sex of baby chicks.

In order to become proficient, an experienced sexer stands next to an apprentice. The apprentice looks at the chick's butt and throws it into the appropriate gender bucket. The teacher gives feedback of "yes" or "no" according to the accuracy of the identification. Imagine you are the apprentice. After weeks of sorting with feedback from your trainer, you will become proficient at the task, despite the fact that you cannot explain how to make the right decision. Intriguing? Unbelievable?

Reading *Incognito* I became fascinated by the hidden workings of the brain. I could not help comparing it to my own experience in medical school when learning about Freud's "id." I remember vividly how my psychiatry professor, an imposing authoritarian but also well-respected authority in the field, tried to explain Freud's concept. Nope. I did not get it. I am still puzzling about the difference between the "Ego" and the "Self." But the idea that stuff was going on in my brain without my knowing and creating havoc without my knowing made total sense.

I recommend that you become a humble, devoted student of the inner working of your brain. I have mentioned neuroplasticity. Instead of dealing with abstract concepts of "Id" and "Self," we get to explore the things under the hood of our car and decide whether or not we will just need a tune up or will need to rebuild the engine!

The take-home message here is that we all store information in the underbelly of the ship, we process information in the underbelly of the ship, and we make decisions based on what is in the underbelly of the ship. If you subscribe to the notion that you are the captain, this might sound a little creepy at first. Who wants to guide an army of mechanics that you know nothing about? But when you think about it, it also opens up a whole new reservoir of options. One is to enjoy getting into the underbelly of the ship simply to have more information available. As the captain, to get back to our analogy, you might want to learn from the mechanics down below. How nice for the captain to have a group of competent engineers he can rely on without knowing anything about the details of who pulls the levers and pushes the buttons.

The body is similar. While it is helpful to know the process and details, you can sometimes simply trust your decisions, even if you cannot explain them. I call this "knowing outside of awareness." People also use the word "intuition" to describe this form of "knowing without knowing." Google defines *intuition* as "the ability to understand something immediately, without the need for conscious reasoning." Close enough!

Throughout the rest of this book, I will ask you to tap into the underbelly of the ship, and sometimes I will encourage you to simply trust your decisions even when you don't know what they are based on. And this is where I want you to link back to accessing your emotions, thoughts, and body sensations as portals to the underbelly of your ship.

The cancer patients I work with are often so relieved when I present this idea of how thoughts and emotions are generated—and at first glance not necessarily or only partly in accordance with external events. Many of them are already all too familiar with their thoughts, body, and emotions having presumably a life of their own and causing hubbub inside. My explanation of the physiological basis relieves them of the burden of "being crazy."

Experiencing something new without understanding what is going on inside the heap of cells can be quite disconcerting and confusing. Sometimes it can seem as if even rebuilding the whole engine will not suffice. In which case learning that an oil change might suffice comes as a big relief.

As I've said, it is a necessary artifice to present thinking, emotion, and body in different chapters, but I can't think of a better way. Where they overlap or interact, I will point this out as to not confuse you. For me it is always about trying to find the most easily relatable and practical way to talk about the complexity of our existence, even if that way is physiologically not perfectly accurate. Let me illustrate with two examples how enmeshed these different components are.

GET USED TO PARADIGM SHIFTS

Just as I have introduced you to the notion that stored information influences our experience and our actions, even though it is not accessible to conscious awareness, I will introduce you to other ideas that might be tempting to reject.

With cancer the emotion that seems most prominent is fear. However, patients will say, "I am anxious." Not "fearful," not "scared" but "anxious." You may have noticed that I never use the word "anxious" or "anxiety" when referring to emotions. I do this both to be aligned with the research on emotion and to address a clinical observation as well. When I ask how patients know that they are anxious, they often pause and say they "just know." They do not know about David Eagleman and *Incognito*, but they "know" anyway. On deeper probing, when they say they feel "anxious," patients describe physical experiences rather than emotions, chest pressure, palpitations, difficulty sleeping, restlessness, irritability, words that by my definition are more closely associated with physical states than emotions.

I want to know exactly what patients are experiencing inside when they say they are "anxious." The more defined the experience, the better our chance of changing it. Anxiety, as it turns out, is often experienced as diffuse, something that feels as if it happens to you rather than something you can take control of. If you find yourself regularly using the word "anxious" to describe yourself, I recommend that you start to pause and examine if you have body correlates to this anxious feeling. It just might be that you are not fearful at all but that you are having physical manifestations of distress.

Another emotion I'd like to reclassify is "worry." Until very recently I would have called "worry" an emotion. In fact I just reviewed a talk I gave in May of 2016, and without hesitation, I called "worry" an emotion. But in reflecting about it while writing this book, I realized that "worry" is mostly a thought-based process. It includes the experience that is associated with unpleasant and concerning thoughts, but the predominant aspect of worry is thought. Worrying without thought content is not possible. Ergo, I can justify reclassifying it (My apologies to the audiences of 2016 and earlier. The principle of "The science of today is the error of tomorrow" obviously applies to me also).

Ultimately the experience "worry" is a mixed process of thought, emotion, and probably other parts of the body and a good illustration of what I called **Thought-Body-Emotion: A Love-Jealousy Triangle** in **Chapter 2**. While I keep longing for purity of body processes, I keep getting confronted with their complex entanglement. In the section on **The Positive Power of Negative Thinking** in **Chapter 4,** you can read in more detail about this complex experience of worry and what to do about it.

Some might argue that it's pointless to split hairs trying to tease apart what constitutes emotion versus thought versus mixed experience. I agree. I do it only to open a window into ourselves. The simplification becomes the skeleton to hang our experiences on, gradually filling in pieces to complete the whole Mensch. It also stimulates discussion, and I hope it helps communication. It is a tool to learn.

CHAPTER 4.

Thinking

We have already covered a lot of ground about thinking in earlier parts of the book. You have learned that thinking is biased, that it often takes place outside of our awareness, feels involuntary, and can be at war with our emotions. Now we'll look at the concept of thought, with the goal of minimizing distress over what I suggest are kinks in thought processes. Remember that thoughts are joined at the hip with body and emotions.

MORE EXERCISES

Let us start with a few short exercises in experiencing thoughts. As with earlier exercises, I ask that you observe and register your experiences while doing the exercise, not just go through the motions of doing it. Do you like it? Do you get annoyed doing the exercise? Do the different exercises evoke different reactions? There is no right or wrong or good or bad. EVERY OBSERVATION GIVES USEFUL INFORMATION! The idea is that you develop a toolbox to create positive experiences while learning how to minimize negative experiences and learn from them. You can jot down what works and what does not. You are creating your own individualized program as you go to accommodate your uniqueness.

Here we go: Take a breath, think about a plant that starts with the letter A, take another breath, think of a plant that starts with the letter B and so on. If you hate plants, pick animals. Be creative! The point is to pick something you like and are familiar with. The answer should come easily, without much thought.

It is important that you take a breath in between every word and focus on breathing out slowly while you work your way through the alphabet. You will learn the why and how it affects your physiology in **Chapter 6** on **Body**. For now I ask that you take my word for it and simply follow the instruction.

If you are someone for whom "breathing stresses me out" (yes, there is such a thing), skip the exercises until you get to the section on **Parasympathetic Exercises** in **Chapter 6** (or take a sneak peek). For the rest of you, keep breathing and thinking about a plant or animal in alphabetical order with at least one breath in between imagined words.

Let's do another exercise. Take a breath and reflect on an emotion you would like to experience right now, then visualize the word for that emotion. If your choice is the word "joyful," you visually create the word "joyful" in front of your mental eye. Once you have decided on your word, visualize it and look at the first letter of the word, in the case of "joyful" you would imagine the letter "j." Take a deep breath again and look at the second letter of the word. Let your eyes rest on it and again take a deep breath. You slowly walk yourself through the word by going from letter to letter and taking a breath in between each letter. If you want to add variety to the exercise, you can also change the color of the letters. If what emerges naturally is black, you can imagine taking one letter and turning it into the color that you associate with a pleasant feeling like joy or relaxation.

In this last exercise, we took advantage of the art of hallucination, seeing something that is not there. But don't worry, in this context, it is healthy. We learned in the beginning that there are individual differences with respect to emotionality, cognition, and physicality. Analogously there are individual differences with respect to ease of creating mental content and enjoyment of mental content. Some people are very visual, others are auditory. Knowing how you process and what mental modalities you enjoy engaging with is helpful when dealing with cancer. As you learn more about your brain, you will be able to use these exercises to your advantage. Sometimes to relax, sometimes to engage with something other than cancer when you wait for your scan or treatment, and sometimes to just have some fun.

If you like numbers and structure or if you don't like letters and plants, give the next exercise a try. Take a breath and start counting backwards from 100 by subtracting serial sevens: 100, take a breath, 93, take a breath, 86, etc.

Reading further will illuminate why I asked you to do these exercises. I hope you remember the core idea in this book that I first presented in Figure 5, which introduced you to Mr. Baldwin. Operating in the "Baldwin paradigm," I could either start with thought, emotion, or body first. I arbitrarily started with thought, partly to accommodate the importance most people give it. Thinking is an important function. Humans pride themselves in their ability to think. It is what presumably sets us apart from other creatures, and many believe that it makes us superior to other creatures.

Thinking is wonderful, but I also believe humans might have gotten a little carried away in their assessment. Not by overrating thinking but by underrating the limitations of thinking and ignoring the importance of emotion and body in the process.

COGNITION, THE GOLDEN CHILD

I don't feel there is fair play when it comes to teaching our children about thought, emotion, and body. Cognition is the favored child, the second we pop out of the womb. Cognition is heavily emphasized in our upbringing. Very early on, reasoning becomes very important, and we get positive feedback for spelling "daddy" at age two but not our emotional expression of crying when falling off the swing. Cartesian dualism at its worst! "Cogito, ergo sum." What about "Sentio, ergo sum?" Interestingly "sentire" in Latin also means "to realize," not just "to feel," as my Latinist son pointed out upon reading a draft of this book. It is a combined sense of realizing and understanding through feeling and perceiving.

I often encourage patients to "realize" through "sentire" rather than "cogitare." But as the result of our cognitively emphasized upbringing, many of us are quite brainy and lose the natural flow and natural access to emotions.

Children freely express their emotions until the sentence, "this is nothing to cry about" eventually leaves its behavioral mark. Joseph LeDoux, an emotion researcher at New York University, reports that after a vital research period on emotions in the first half of the 20th century, research on cognition got the upper hand as cognition was viewed as a computer-like process and thus objective and that a "dark cloud of subjectivity hung over the topic of emotions" (LeDoux, 2000).

I have introduced you to some limitations of thinking early to tickle your interest for a paradigm shift in your approach to your own thinking. I have also presented information about the relevance of distress in cancer patients. And I have hinted that the two don't make good bed partners, which as a cancer patient is a problem. How you think when you are distressed, which is pretty much the whole time when dealing with cancer, does not serve you well. There are many ways thought can get messed up, but the one you definitely need to understand is how it gets messed up in the presence of distress.

THOUGHTS UNDER DURESS

When humans are distressed, their capacity for logical thinking is impaired. We revert back to animal cognition. The stressful force of cancer constitutes duress and we resemble more a hyena in the savanna than Einstein in his brightest moment. We regress to the abilities we had before cognition evolved for humans. Cancer patients are often puzzled by the disconnect between their ability to reason and their inability to act on reasoning, but it makes perfect sense if you look at what distress does to cognition, as you are about to read in more detail.

Bridging the disconnect between the rational and the emotional brain is an important asset to functioning effectively. It will decrease your distress, so you don't act like an ostrich putting your head in the sand but optimize your thought ability to make good choices when it matters most. You want your thinking at your best to make the best possible choices for your treatment and your health.

THOUGHTS ARE A SUBSET OF COGNITION

Thinking is a subcategory of cognition. I often see the words interchangeably used. To stay within the framework that thoughts serve as "a window into our incognito existence," I will mostly use the word "thinking."

But cognition is more than thinking. Science on cognition is complex, but a little crash course will help you better understand your own thinking and how to use it to your advantage.

In your exchange with the world and yourself, you have to be able to perceive information, process it, retain it, and retrieve it. Cognition is also the process of producing focus, attention, and concentration. Memory is responsible for storage and retrieval of information. You will hear the term "executive function" as well. This refers to your ability to plan and take goal-oriented action, a fundamental feature when you deal with cancer. Another aspect called "inhibition" is the ability to inhibit thoughts so you can selectively pay attention to relevant information. The latter is definitely something cancer patients struggle with. You become easily flooded with irrelevant thoughts. The important take-home message here is that cognitive functions are impaired with distress (Shields et al., 2016), and you have to make accommodations for this.

But distress is just one experience that messes with cognition. Cancer and its treatment affect cognition on various levels beyond distress. If you think your cognition is affected, your thinking is not as sharp, your brain foggy, your memory a disaster, and you feel it is not caused by distress, turn to the section on **Cognitive Function** in **Chapter 13** on **Survivorship** where you will get to know Shelli Kesler and her devotion to helping patients with cognitive difficulty as a result of cancer. The latter is commonly referred to as "chemobrain," even though it is not just chemotherapy that causes this problem.

NAGGING THOUGHTS AND THE PRINCIPLE OF RIGIDITY

Dealing with stressful thought is an important focus in my work and unfortunately also one of the hardest nuts to crack. Cancer can be a very thought-driven affair. Recurring thoughts of funeral arrangements after a cancer cure are not uncommon. These thoughts worsen the distress of cancer. We briefly touched on how distress distorts thinking, but the reverse is also true: distorted thinking is quite stressful, too.

I hope you recall Figure 5, which by now is hopefully photographed into your brain. Negative thoughts induce distress. How and what we think about the stressor can be as stress evoking to emotions and the body as the event itself.

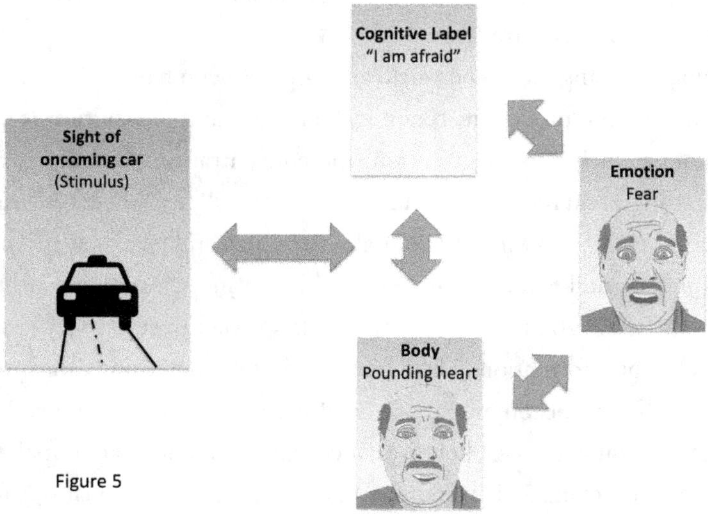

Figure 5

I want you to pause and take in that sentence again. Having a stressful thought is stressful on the body. This sentence reinforces the content from the section about the intimate relationship between events and how we humans process them. I am referring back to earlier in the book when I said that if thoughts could just be—without causing havoc to other parts of the body—we would not have to change them.

Many patients are familiar with the distress that arises with thoughts that cancer might return. The thought "My cancer will come back" can evoke a more stressful body and emotional response than the cancer recurrence itself. Many of you think of recurrence while you are being treated and have a chance at cure. Are you aware of how that introduces distress to your existence? And it is not just patients who think about recurrence after cancer. As you know, your friends and family sometimes worry about it more than you do.

We have established that our brains generate thoughts that don't seem helpful, but some of these thoughts can be obnoxiously persistent. Patients often describe their thinking as "fixated, hijacked, intrusive."

"I don't want to think the thought, and it thinks itself anyway." Jill Smolowe, an award-winning journalist and author, wrote an eloquent, moving, and succinct account of her experience with her husband's leukemia and later death. In *Four Funerals and a Wedding*, she describes "that a deepening anxiety gradually straightjacketed my thinking" and "that nonstop discussions about Joe's illness might mire my thoughts in a repetitive groove." She experienced thinking as overpowering, rigid, and insurmountable. As we discussed, most people can easily relate to having a response to an external stressor, but it takes some convincing that our thinking about the event and how it relates to us can evoke as much of a stress response as the event itself.

This is an example of inhibition of thoughts not working. We are thinking what we do not want to think. Why is this? What can you do about it? Read on.

THE PHYSIOLOGY OF THINKING AND EVOLUTION

Since thoughts are such an important aspect of the cancer experience, I want to open your mind about thinking and cognition in general. *The Organized Mind* by Daniel J. Levitin, a retired neuroscientist at McGill University in Canada, is an eloquently written book that educates us about the brain and in particular about cognition and thoughts. Levitin describes how the brain perceives, processes, stores, and retrieves information and describes the many flaws of the mind that prevent us from effectively functioning. His sentence, "the evolved structure of the brain is haphazard and disjointed, and incorporates multiple systems, each of which has a mind of its own" is very much relevant to patients with cancer.

With cancer patients, thinking tends to take on a life of its own. Instead of the organizational systems in the brain working synergistically, patients experience disorganization. Thoughts like "I am looking forward to my son's wedding" easily coexist with, "I am so sad that I won't be at my son's wedding." This thinking takes place regardless of your cancer status. You can be cured or have been told that you will have to adjust to living with cancer in your body, and the thoughts don't seem to correlate with your health status. These thoughts are associated with whatever state your body is in in any given second. Distressed or not distressed. Not only did evolution not deliver us a perfectly developed brain, it falls apart when we are stressed!

Levitin compares the evolutionary development of the brain to an old house. You add things to the house and remodel as you need them, one at a time. You usually do not come up with the perfect design when you first build the house, or even if you do, you might not have the money to execute it. You start with the air conditioner unit in one bedroom and eventually you might be financially sound enough to air condition the whole house. But you probably won't remove the single unit from the bedroom. Whatever image we use, I interpret his description as a way to explain that our brain might not always function in our best interest. To have the single air conditioner unit run after you air condition the whole house does not make sense, but it's a remnant from an earlier phase of building. My illustration of thinking about funeral arrangements after a cancer cure would be an example of this.

What exactly is the brain doing when it has thoughts about making funeral arrangements after your doctor has told you that you are cured? Is there a purpose to this kind of thinking, or is it simply a kind of evolutionary holdover, a malfunctioning of the brain when distressed? Why would the brain think a thought that is not based in the reality of one's health? Neuroscience sheds some light on this conundrum. "Humankind cannot bear much reality," T. S. Eliot observed, and "humankind" loves to tell stories to tolerate the unbearable reality.

According to Levitin, the right brain is the fact tracker and the left brain is responsible for "making order out of chaos, for making sense of things in the world that don't always add up." The only problem? The left brain makes stuff up. It confabulates. It lies to suit the purpose of making sense. Usually people don't give that fact much thought, but the Covid-19 pandemic drives the point home.

Reporting about how humans deal with uncertainty in the context of the Covid pandemic, Stephen Hinshaw, a professor of psychology at UC Berkeley, was quoted in the *San Francisco Chronicle* (Kost, 2021) as saying, "We create narratives to understand ourselves and the world. And by definition, a narrative, a story, has a beginning, middle, and an end. Without an end, though it's harder to craft a narrative and harder to get some resolution." The technical term for this is cognitive closure, but in more simple terms, if you don't like your reality, you fill it with your own fiction. Even though Professor Hinshaw used the example in the context of the Covid-19 pandemic, the lack of cognitive closure is very similar with cancer.

As a human, you always have to consider this. Whether this will be an evolutionary survival advantage needs to be seen. As Levitin points out, "evolution doesn't design things and it doesn't build systems—it settles on a system that, historically, conveyed a survival benefit (and if a better way comes along, it will adopt that)."

THOUGHT SEIZURES

Levitin and Eagleman teach us that the brain is a vast storage container of which most information is not part of our awareness and often not retrievable, or at least difficult to retrieve; it is built like a haphazardly thrown-together house and it has limited processing speed, and when it generates thought, it often confabulates. Great! Smolowe describes the repetitious, unwanted appearance of thought. She calls it hijacked and grooved; I call it "thought seizure."

Seizures are the result of an "episode of abnormal electrical activity in the brain." People understand that abnormal electrical activity in the brain can lead to involuntary muscle contractions but at first seem puzzled when I declare that thoughts are no different from muscles. Thoughts as a result of involuntary electrical activity are no different to me than muscles twitching as the result of involuntary electrical activity. Just a different location and different process but nevertheless the same principle.

This is in part why I am not rigidly opposed to prescribing benzodiazepines during cancer treatment. Many patients get them anyway as part of their anti-nausea regimen. What a wonderful way to catch two birds with one stone. I have worked with cancer patients who experience benzodiazepines as antidepressants, which makes perfect sense because of the close association of thoughts and emotions. When we lighten thoughts, we will lift mood. If a long-accumulated reservoir of thoughts can impact your emotions and body, imagine what mayhem repetitious unwanted thoughts can cause you. Time to figure out how to deal with this seizure-style thinking.

THE BRAIN, THE SLOWPOKE

Levitin's book comes to the rescue. In addition to confabulating, he explains that the brain appears to be rather slow at processing conscious information. From his review of the available research, he tells us that the conscious mind seems to have a processing capacity of 120 bits per second, not that much when you consider that the average person watches five hours of TV per day, which constitutes the equivalent of twenty gigabytes of audio-video images to process. As someone who barely knows the difference between bits and bytes, I probably did the conversion wrong, but according to an online converter, this would be 160,000,000,000 bits. Poor brain! Reading about this limited processing speed for the first time sounded like an obstacle to human functionality, but then it dawned on me that this very slowness offers us a way out of rigid thought seizures! Bear with me here on these details. I want to make sure they help the exercises make sense.

Have you ever noticed that people are often a little absentminded on the phone? If they are surfing the web while talking with you, which they often are—I will not go into the "Miss Manners" aspect of the behavior—they are obviously exceeding their 120 bits. I have tested this on myself. I can do menial tasks, like chopping carrots or watering the yard, while attempting a sensible conversation on the phone, but that is the extent of my ability to multitask.

I always thought of my brain as somewhat of a loser for not being a multitasking genius until I read *Deep Work* by Cal Newport. Newport posits that uni-tasking, the ability to focus on one thing, is our real superpower. Now I carry my brain's ability for depth like a badge of pride. And I see that what is necessary is that we pack *quality* into our 120 bits per second rather than multitudes! All this deep thinking inspired a helpful clinical exercise.

Remember the exercises at the beginning of **Chapter 4** when I had you think of animals or plants in alphabetical order and take breath in between words? Or when I asked you to think of an emotion you wanted to feel and had you visualize the word for it? I developed these exercises precisely to take advantage of our limited processing capacity. These techniques allow you to "ungroove" thought patterns, even if they were generated a million times before. We are revisiting "Neurons wire together if they fire together" but with the opposite aim.

"If we can get those neurons that fire stupid thoughts to stop firing, they will stop wiring."

Those measly 120 bits per second might sound like the capacity of a mouse brain, but they are in fact our ally. If we give the brain *something else to do*, we can start to shrink the shitty thought wires! The presumed flaw becomes an asset!

Now start thinking of flowers starting with the letter A...

Many exercises you encounter in this book take advantage of the fact that the human brain is such a slowpoke. But remember this is just the conscious mind. The brain also processes outside of our awareness constantly and in addition to the 120 bits per second. Remember incognito.

THOUGHT STACKING

I propose that you use this processing speed (or rather processing slowness) to your advantage by crowding out stuff that you don't want to think about. And not just crowd it out but slowly dismantle its neuronal structure. There is another style of thinking in addition to "thought seizures" for which that works. I call it "thought stacking." Rather than random thoughts popping like corn in the pan, they build momentum off one another like a runaway train. One negative thought stacks onto the next.

We're dealing not just with a series of negative thoughts but with thoughts the next of which is worse than the one before. "I did not present myself well during the interview" is followed by "I will never get this job" is followed by "I will lose my house" is followed by "My wife will leave me." Some people call this thought sequencing *catastrophizing*.

If you are someone for whom every thought is worse than the previous one, you probably get plenty of advice about not catastrophizing. This style of thinking is very common with distress. But rather than get disappointed that you don't seem able to follow the well-meant sapient advice of your family and friends, try any of the exercises in this book and interrupt the thought stacks. Not catastrophizing might be a tall order, but crowding out the cascade of thoughts is something you can do.

METACOGNITION

Another aspect of thinking is called metacognition. It is the process of having thoughts about thoughts. While this can be an interesting pastime when we feel well, distress can turn these thoughts about thoughts quite nasty. Negative and critical (as in self-critical and judgmental, not as in critiquing and evaluating) runaway train thinking is an ineffective way to conquer thought with thought. "You should not think that way. You know that these thoughts are not helpful" is a setup for disaster. "This cancer will kill me," and the next thought is "I should not think that way, I need to think positively." We think thoughts about thoughts. The same way I recommend reframing "catastrophizing," I want to encourage you to disengage from metacognition as much as you can while you are sick (more on this throughout, particularly as many exercises are geared towards this goal). Most of us simply do not have the ability to think ourselves out of our thoughts. When you catch yourself hearing yourself think "should," it's really an invitation working on doing something else. Literally anything is a better alternative.

MONKEY MIND

The term *monkey mind* has gained some currency in recent years. You will often find it used to describe erratic thinking, popcorn style, or runaway train style or metacognition. I don't think we do monkeys justice here because only humans have a monkey mind. Monkeys don't exert that kind of erratic thought; they are more preoccupied with how to get the next orange. But as I am sure you know, it is not fun, particularly if you do this type of thinking as a cancer patient. It can take you down some very dark alleys. There is a whole science debate dedicated to repetitive negative thought content, but the concepts you will encounter the most are *worrying* and *rumination*, the former usually defined as repetitive, uncontrollable thinking about feared future events (which many of you are very familiar with) and the latter as repetitive, aversive, and uncontrollable self-focused thought that centers on past negative experiences (Szkodny & Newman, 2019). It doesn't matter what word you use, as long as you realize it does not serve you well. A negative thinking style and a repetitious focus on distress of any kind does not do the brain any good.

I can recommend several books that talk about this phenomenon: *Monkey Mind* by Daniel Smith is one. *I Wish I Could Be There* by Allen Shawn is another movingly written self-reflection on the topic of thoughts taking on a life of their own and the havoc they can create. Importantly these books are not just about thinking gone haywire, they all deal with what happens as a result of extensive negative thinking.

What I want to stress is this: Don't get stuck in the chicken-and-egg question. Is negative thinking affecting body and emotions, or is distress causing negative thoughts? Both are true. Remember our discussion of the bidirectional connection of thought, emotion, and body? These books offer impressive examples of the impact of detrimental thinking on body and emotions and the scientific literature also provides ample evidence. The bottom line is rumination contributes to the development of depressed mood and affects executive functioning (Yang et al., 2017).

THOUGHTS AND ACTIONS

Having useless thoughts per se is not the problem. Thinking them is a waste of your time. But the fact that thoughts can have a negative impact on other parts of the body, this takes them beyond just time wasters. An additional component is that acting on them can get us in trouble. We often live by our own beliefs, even if it is to our disadvantage. People call it self-sabotaging. I would not use that expression; I call it acting on conditioned thoughts.

If you believe that "success can only come through hard work," then there is a good chance that you act in ways that are consistent with that belief. Imagine you believe that "I cannot die before my children are launched into independence." There is a good chance you will either drive your children crazy expediting their launching or feel discouraged if they do not act on your belief. Often there is a cost-benefit analysis involved in the thought process. The cost of going on with life, to use the previous belief as an example, might be pain, arduous treatment, and sleepless nights, but the benefit is being around for your children as long as possible to help them become independent. I have had many patients whose main purpose was to be there for the children to grow up.

But thoughts and beliefs don't just guide our actions, they also prevent us from acting. If you think, for example, "I cannot play this piece of music unless I play it perfectly," there is a good chance you will not play the music at all as only few people have the skill to play a piece without a slip. Sometimes it can even be thoughts of parents or other relatives that can influence how we experience ourselves.

Karen was diagnosed with metastatic cancer at a young age. She was very pragmatic about treatment but felt conflicted since her mother had approached her own illness many years earlier in a very different way. Her mother's sentence that "I do not want any poison in my body" lived in Karen as, "Am I wrong to have opted for high-dose chemotherapy?"

I want you to examine your thinking for thoughts that might prevent you from taking helpful action. Karen didn't feel comfortable with her choice of chemotherapy until she realized that her mother's belief system interfered with her own actions.

MORE PRACTICE

Let us do the practical exercises again to see if you experience them differently now that you know about your mouse brain processing speed. Does it help you to understand that the success of the exercises is related to our 120 bits per second limitation? (In **Chapter 6**, on **Body**, you will learn the details of why it is important to breathe and how. As I said before, if you are someone who struggles to breathe and feels stressed by it, skip the exercise section for now or do the exercise without the conscious breath in between.)

Take a breath, think about a plant that starts with the letter A, take another breath, think of a plant that starts with the letter B, and so on. There are numerous variations to this theme. Get creative! Don't forget the slow breath in between.

And here, another repeat: Take a breath and visualize a word that represents an emotion you would like to experience right now. If it is the word "joyful," visually create the word "joyful" in front of your mental eye. Once you have decided on the word, visualize it and look at its first letter. Now take a deep breath and look at the second letter of the word. Let your eyes rest on it and again take a deep breath. Slowly walk yourself through the word by going from letter to letter and taking a breath in between each letter. If you want to add variety to the exercise, you can also change the color of the letters. If what emerges naturally is black, you can imagine taking one letter and turning it into the color that you associate with a pleasant feeling, like joy or relaxation. And just to give the exercise a different flavor, try to do it with the word "healing."

And here again the version for the number people among you: Take a breath and start counting backwards from 100 by subtracting serial sevens: 100, take a breath, 93, take a breath, 86 etc.

Critical readers will notice that some of these practices are not strictly "thought" exercises but involve other functions of cognition, but the devil for a change is not in the details. It doesn't matter. The bottom line is as long as you breathe and give your brain 120 bits of non-stressful activity, you will be reasonably content.

This last suggestion is one of the few that can leave me in a heated discussion with my patients. "So you want me to distract myself from my cancer-related thoughts?" is a common question. Some of you might even call the suggestion an instruction to avoid, at which point I turn on my most charming beagle eyes.

"If anything is a distraction, it is spending time with negative thought content. These thoughts are a distraction from living your life" is how I counter when necessary. If I still meet resistance, I release my avalanche of research evidence about worry and rumination, the thought stacking of repetitious negative beliefs, that I mentioned a few pages back.

No, when we give our brain alternatives to negative, distressful thought, we are not distracting. We are giving a break to the parts of the brain that are engaged in stressful activity! Not only do I recommend eliminating judgmental language, I also want you to optimize your choice of thought and words based on the physiology of the body. I am asking you to shift your focus from one thought to another less stressful or even pleasant but at least a neutral thought or activity.

FOCUS

You might say my exercises force you into a focused state. But this begs the question: what, exactly, is focus? Focus is not solely a thought process but involves many other aspects of cognition and perception. I discuss it in the chapter on thoughts because many of us have difficulty not focusing on negative thought.

You'll recall Winnie Gallagher from the first two chapters. Gallagher, author of *Rapt: Attention and the Focused Life* writes that science proves that "You cannot always be happy but you can almost always be focused, which is the next best thing." It is an encouraging motto. Gallagher encourages you to focus on health rather than illness and to battle your negativity bias. She shares the insight that "this disease wanted to monopolize my attention, but as much as possible, I would focus on my life instead."

As you know, this is easier said than done. When Gallagher wanted to pay attention to her life, she had to learn *not* to pay attention to how her thoughts about cancer made her feel like shit. But how do you do that? The most common recommendation you will get is to have "positive thoughts." You will get bombarded with recommendations to think positively.

If you have the ability to do that, go for it. But if you are like me, whose brain has a propensity to succumb to negative thoughts with much more ease than positive ones, I propose alternatives.

I want you to assess your focus. Are you focusing on illness? Are you focusing on thoughts other than illness, and are any of these thoughts helpful? Figure 6 presents an image that will walk you through what ultimately constitutes four choices.

Figure 6

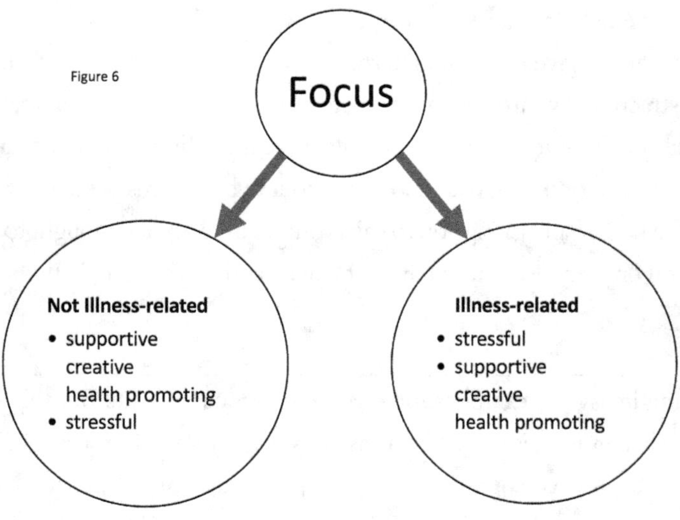

Looking at this figure, you can see that both thinking about illness and thinking about something else can be beneficial—or not. Please don't interpret this to mean I'm telling you not to focus on illness. I am asking you to develop awareness to *focus on what is helpful to your health*, whether you are thinking about your illness or something else. I also want you to notice that you don't see the words "positive" and "negative" in this algorithm. The algorithm is an invitation to assess whether the thoughts are useful or pleasant regardless of whether they are positive, negative, or related to illness. They are just thoughts to notice.

INHIBITION

Earlier I mentioned the cognitive function of "inhibition." Cancer often challenges the ability to inhibit thoughts in order to selectively pay attention to relevant information. You are at times flooded with irrelevant thoughts. Particularly at night, when the brain is left to its own thoughts, you don't have the same options for focused thought. Better inhibition would be nice, but in the stillness of the night, there's often nothing else to fill the 120 bits! At night thoughts can often take on an overly worried, even paranoid flavor and meta-cognition runs rampant. Those are times when a focused, relaxing approach might work better than letting your thoughts wander.

There are other situations where thoughts don't get suppressed that you wished would be. In meditation and guided imagery classes, for example, you will often be instructed to imagine a safe place or see yourself walking on a beach. While this is a wonderful suggestion in theory, there are plenty of people who will realize during the exercise that they do not have a safe place to connect to in their mind, which in itself can be quite traumatic. Alternatively, while you create pleasant images of walking on the beach and might even be able to hallucinate the warmth of the sun and the texture of the sand, you are also at risk for intrusive negative thought content. Imagine taking a visual stroll, and all of a sudden you have an image of a loved one with whom you spent time on this particular beach but whom you lost. Not fun! The pleasant effect of the guided imagery will be annihilated, and you will immediately connect to unpleasant emotions that are associated with that image or memory. Remember that thought and emotion are bidirectionally associated and connected. And also remember that inhibition of thoughts does not happen easily, particularly when you are distressed.

THE PENSIEVE

It is not just machination about the creation of thought that I'm asking you to be aware of, so you don't stumble into an excavation pit of your partially remodeled brain house. I have discussed the evolution of thought-generating brain structures, thought's speed (or lack thereof), the interrelatedness with emotion and distress, and I have suggested how you can use some of the presumed flaws to your advantage. Another topic relevant to cancer patients is storage and retrieval.

I am still wrapping my head around the notion that I introduced you to earlier that every conscious experience might be stored. The brain, a hard drive. I am not sure whether it is fortunate or unfortunate that most of this information is not retrievable. Ask yourself if you would want that ability. Sometimes it would be wonderful to be able to retrieve by choice, but depending on what you experienced in your life, you might happily forgo the option.

Remember Professor Albus Dumbledore from the Harry Potter books? His Pensieve holds your memories and helps you tap into them. Both Harry and Dumbledore get illuminating insight, but at times the process looks unpleasant. I encourage you to keep that piece of information present. It cuts both ways, good or bad.

When you experience something that you cannot grasp, rather than assume you are nuts, consider that we have an "incognito" process involved. I have already advocated for getting to know "incognito" better to be more effective with your brain, and I will keep advocating for it. Remember the window into yourself? Emotions, thoughts, and physical sensations!

MEMORY

In order to understand the "storage container of thought," we will have to deal with memory itself. It is another aspect of cognition related to thought that people—with or without cancer—have problems with. Details of memory research are beyond the focus of this book, but I do want to address the cancer-relevant parts.

Remembering is a function of cognition, which is often impaired as part of distress and cancer treatment, but to remember is also an important aspect for cancer patients. You might have noticed since your diagnosis that you more often reminisce. Reminiscence comes with thoughts about the past. Sometimes it comes with a desire to process the past. Those motivations are laudable, but I want to caution you about the desire for accuracy of memory. Memory does not always constitute events and facts from the past you can simply retrieve from storage. What we retrieve has a tendency to change over time.

The parts of memory you can consciously recall or "declare" are also called declarative memory. You will also see it called "explicit" memory, even though that term is technically not quite accurate. But it does not matter. The important thing is not to get hung up on accuracy when you reminisce as this can cost you precious loss of time and a considerable amount of distress.

You will also need to differentiate declarative memory from emotional memory, which is very important for cancer patients but a totally different ballgame altogether. The thing to remember is that declarative is memory is often inaccurate.

Try to minimize arguments with others about the accuracy of your thoughts about the past. "I remember exactly that you were mean to me on October 17th, 1998" will not take you to helpful places. Not only do we tell ourselves stories to make sense of the world, but even when we think we are accurately retrieving memory from storage, we often are not.

How information gets stored when you are distressed is also important for cancer patients. Traumatic memories—and cancer often creates traumatic memories—seem to be burned into the brain differently, often quite accurately, which is different from the type of storage I just described above. Bessel Van der Kolk, whom I mentioned earlier, uses a simple illustration in his book *The Body Keeps the Score*. He reminds the reader that most of you probably remember where you were on September 11th, 2001 but have no recollection of what you did on September 10th. So on one hand, your brain is not that great at remembering, but recollections of traumatic experiences can be quite accurate. The point about memory to take away is that its accuracy can cover the whole range from super accurate to fabricated, with you unfortunately not knowing the difference. So you have to be thoughtful about how you approach memory.

THOUGHTS ARE STAND-INS FOR NEEDS

I have suggested that you can shift your focus when you don't like your thoughts, but I also encourage you to explore your thoughts, unless doing so creates too much distress. I ultimately will not be able to answer whether the obsessive nature of human thoughts is an evolutionary error or has purpose, but my clinical experience is that thoughts often express needs, wishes, and desires or discontent about the absence of fulfilled needs and wishes. So as an alternative to giving the brain 120 bits per second of activity to banish some thoughts as if they were mutinous renegades, we can explore them instead.

Reflecting on the color of the flower arrangements you'd like at your funeral at some undetermined time in the future is a thought process, yes, but a pretty moot one unless death is near, no? Unfortunately some patients who are cured think about funeral arrangements also. In Figure 6, I suggested that if your focus on thoughts does not produce anything helpful, you might focus on something else. If the brain is so haphazardly built and unreliable in its production of thought, why explore what, at least at first glance, doesn't make sense? Right. So what if we dug deeper to explore what might be motivating you to reflect on that particular future?

I believe this particular thought is not so much about the actual planning but represents, for example, a desire for certainty, predictability, and control. Thoughts about funeral arrangements can represent wanting certainty. The act of exploring whether the thought presents an unmet need takes fear out of the picture and I believe helps you tap into your Pensieve more accurately than reasoning.

The simplest version of my "Pensieve exercise" usually puzzles people. An illustration would be, "I am churning thoughts before I fall asleep to fulfill my need for x." You take a behavior you want to change, in this example wanting to sleep rather than think, and speculate about its motive. But instead of thinking about it, you let the body retrieve a word. "First word, single word, noun" is my instruction. After some objection usually having to do with wanting to analyze the process, most people surrender to the process of body association with a funny look on their face. And most often, the word that pops up is relevant to the person's life.

When Jay, a busy contractor, did the exercise on churning thought before sleep, his word was "completion." He was intrigued. It helped him realize that thinking before going to sleep fulfilled the purpose of mentally closing out all of the business transactions of the day. When he shifted that activity to the sofa with a writing pad after coming home from work, his wish for completion was fulfilled. When he went to bed later, the desire did not interfere with falling asleep.

You will read more throughout the book about this need-based concept with **Chapter 8** exclusively devoted to it, but I want to give you a flavor with an additional example of how you can take advantage of your stored information and try to make sense of the thought-seizing, thought-stacking brain under duress. Jay wanted "completion," and most every human seems to want certainty.

As it turns out, humans are not good at uncertainty. Nothing has brought that home more acutely than the pandemic. Usually we are not confronted with holding uncertainty in our awareness, but the recent pandemic made it apparent how humans struggle with uncertainty as Professor Hinshaw had commented earlier. It is easier for the world at large to ignore the uncertainty struggle of cancer patients, even though there are millions of them, but all of a sudden, everybody in the world was in the same pandemic boat and had to confront uncertainty.

Certainty is a basic human longing, but uncertainty is a hallmark of cancer. At the time of diagnosis, you don't know what the treatment will look like, during treatment you don't know what to expect, and after treatment you may worry that the cancer will come back. But instead of learning to live with the fact of uncertainty (hello, fact recorder right brain), you create what I call a "fictitious but possible" reality (hello, confabulating left brain) just to satisfy your desire for certainty. Thinking about funeral arrangements after a cancer cure may at first seem odd, but it fulfills the desire for certainty. Thoughts about choosing the color of the funeral announcement cards also represent a form of control, but thoughts about the uncertainty of illness or death feel intrusively disconcerting. Since certainty is such a common need, you can always explore if your stressful thoughts might represent that need.

THE POSITIVE POWER OF NEGATIVE THINKING

I snagged the heading for this section from a book title by Julie K. Norem, a professor at Wellesley College. She has contemplated a possible function of negative thinking. Could it in fact be that negative thought is a good thing? My clinical and personal experience says hardly ever. I am sure you have caught yourself feeling stuck in thoughts in reaction to something that happened in the past or are ruminating about something that could happen in the future. Did that style of thinking help you? Let's see what her research has to say.

Norem studied a subset of people whom her teacher Nancy Cantor had previously coined *Defensive Pessimists*. Defensive pessimists focus on potentially bad outcomes; they also carefully consider all possible outcomes, and they picture how they could fix things if something went wrong. They seem to feel that considering what can go wrong helps them to prepare. In a series of elegantly designed experiments, Norem demonstrated that defensive pessimism "encompasses an entire process by which negative thinking transforms anxiety into action."

According to Norem, thinking and preparing in a reaction to a future task is a coping strategy to decrease fear. When the actual task that evoked worry, like giving a presentation, comes around, you won't feel the fear and perform just fine. Norem states that the "mental rehearsal resembles a coping imagery technique that sports psychologist use to prepare athletes for upcoming performances." If you deprive defensive pessimists of that preparation thought coping strategy and force them into positive thinking or stress reduction through meditation, they in fact perform worse on specific tasks, like dart throwing (Norem, 2001).

And Norem is not the only one researching the possible benefits of negative thinking. Szabó and Lovibond (2002) report that almost half of naturally occurring worrying thoughts are in the category of problem solving and suggested that "worry consists largely of attempted problem solving."

"One possible mechanism of pathological worry," they write, "may be a failure to bring problem solving to a satisfactory conclusion." Basically, following the motto, "let me think until my head blows up and a solution will occur."

Could this style of thinking help you? I am on board if the thoughts produce a result, a solution, or have a soothing component. But I rarely see that to be the case in my patients. You can assess your thinking in terms of producing a solution or its effectiveness on calming your nerves. There is also an important distinction between these studies and the issues cancer patients experience with worrying, which is a difference in content. Worrying about an evaluation for promotion is about a specific, defined event at a specific time in the future, while the worries about cancer neither have a specific date nor a specific content and often drift to the scary vagueness of death, loss, and suffering.

If you identify as a *defensive pessimist* and happen to develop cancer, take into account that you naturally will want to apply your problem-solving-future-thinking-worst-case-scenario-preventing self. In the case of cancer, however, these familiar practices might not be effective. We tend to apply what we are used to and best at rather than what's applicable and effective. My hope is that learning different techniques in this book will expand your repertoire of choices.

In your assessment about the usefulness of thinking as a coping strategy, always be aware of rumination. I mentioned rumination earlier in this chapter. It often constitutes simply repeating thoughts, and often very stressful ones at that, without presenting a solution or taking action. And I get support for that notion from science. "Rumination will do you no good. You will consider your problems unsolvable, you will have little motivation to implement change, and you won't reach out to your friends. Do you really want that?" (Ordaz et al., 2017)

I found an additional piece of information that made me wonder if it might be the distinguishing factor explaining why the pessimistic thinking might work for preparing talks or math tests but not for cancer. Szabó and Lovibond (2006) made the interesting observation that individuals who rated their worry episodes as more uncontrollable were less likely to engage in problem solving and were also more likely to keep worrying until they became distracted by an external event.

Uncontrollability is a component that many patients describe in their experience with cancer. As long as patients feel they can control the cancer by being proactive in treatment, they often do reasonably well despite enduring miserable side effects, but as soon as treatment is done, the feeling that the cancer might come back or progress leaves a sense of uncontrollability.

The fear of giving a talk or failing at throwing darts or a conversation with your boss is ultimately very different from the experience cancer.

Now that we've established that excessive worrying decreases your chances at effective problem solving, I want you to make sure to differentiate worrying thoughts from thinking about illness in a productive way as I mentioned in the section on focus. It is important that you use thinking about your illness as part of the process of finding solutions for it. You might want to contemplate your illness to find peace with it. But what you don't want to do is focus on your illness in ways that create distress rather than solutions. Worry is an aspect of thinking you have to be vigilant to catch in its early stages before it gets out of hand.

Another aspect of worrying is that we use it in order to buffer unpleasant feelings. But does it work? There is research that supports the idea that worrying about a negative outcome reduces the disappointment should the negative outcome come to pass. But the study was done in a situation where an event had already happened (waiting for the result of the bar exam), and people were examined while waiting for the result, which is very different from the fear that something *might* happen in the future but also has a chance of n*ot* happening.

Let's look at the study anyway, as it might assist with other aspects of your life, even if it is not completely representative of your situation with cancer. Law students who had taken the bar exam had to wait for a few weeks for the results (Hoffman, *New York Times*, November 2, 2015). The worriers were positively surprised when they passed the bar but not shattered when they flunked because they had braced themselves for the failure. This is interesting and relatable but does not exactly mirror the situation for most patients with cancer. With cancer you are not waiting to hear about an already determined outcome but are scared of the unpredictability of the future, like progression or recurrence. Unlike the law students, your outcome has not been determined yet. Whether or not they are worried about it ahead of time, most people with cancer are shattered if their worst-case scenario comes true.

If you are a worrier and can test if your worrisome thinking lowers your angst or enables you to produce solutions, I do not want to discourage you. I believe wholeheartedly that each person's path to well-being is unique. But I do strenuously urge you to assess whether your thinking style induces distress, and if it does, to do something else, no matter what or how. If you feel that your brain is just churning out unproductive thought, you are better off engaging your conscious mind's processing capacity of 120 bits per second with something else.

Observe when repetitious and negative thought content takes place and assess if there is any benefit from it without paying the price of distress. If not it is probably not worthwhile. Remember Levitin's description of the fact-tracking part of the brain and the confabulating brain that tries to make sense of things. We invent stories to make sense of the world. Those stories, however, don't always help us solve our problems and are not always based in our actual reality.

POSITIVE THINKING

The discussion about the downside or potential benefits of negative thought naturally leads to a discussion about positive thinking. I already demonstrated in **Chapter 2** how interconnected thought, emotion, and body are, and I won't retract that here. But let's look at the topic in more depth. I want to talk about positive thought in the same breath and for the same reason I talked about negative thoughts, which is the potential to create distress, albeit for different reasons.

With negative thinking, it is the thought itself that can cause distress, with positive thinking it is the stress around the inability to create it, not the thought itself. If you are someone who creates positive thoughts with ease, enjoy them and skip this section, otherwise read on.

The branch of psychology that deals with this phenomenon is called "Positive Psychology," which you've probably heard of as the popular literature is plastered with it. As you can imagine from the name, positive psychology focuses on positivity. Positive thoughts, positive emotions. "Creation of positive thoughts" is central to the several billion-dollar industry of positive psychology. Most everybody acknowledges that negative thought is rarely useful and believes in the value of thinking positively. Sure, but I think we all know that it is easier said than done. Later in the book, you'll find a considerable proportion of **Chapter 7** devoted to **Positive Psychology** (an expansion from just positive thought), but I'll start you with some suggestions here. And there are some pitfalls with focus on positivity that I need you to be aware of.

First of all, let's differentiate *focus* on positive thought from *creation* of positive thoughts. If you have positive thought content that you can easily concentrate on, wonderful, but if you must labor to create positive thought or get stressed by the process, there's little point to it, and in fact its purpose is defeated. It's important that you accommodate your personal thinking style and not try to fit a round peg into a square hole.

I have seen many people get quite distressed by the difficulty of creating positive thought content. It throws them straight back to their days in school, when they did not want to suck at something. They feel like failures when they can't easily create positive thoughts; it's like a performance failure. And it is not just a frustration with not being able to create positive content easily; it is also the fear of the negative impact of negative thoughts. Some people understandably interpret the push to think positively to mean, "If I have negative thoughts, my cancer will come back." How's that for some negative thought content? I absolutely don't want you to get stressed if you have difficulty in creating positive thoughts. While I advocate the creation of positive thought content, if you can do it with ease, don't sweat it if you struggle with it. Please.

But it is not just performance stress that matters with positive thinking. While I don't agree with some of Carl Gustav Jung's life-style and professional actions, his statement that "the conscious mind allows itself to be trained like a parrot but the unconscious does not" is spot on (Jung, 1953). You can repeat a conscious mantra like, "I am a successful person," but if unconsciously you believe that you are a loser, you will have conflicting voices to deal with. Jung's insight is another reason why positive thinking is not as easy as some people make it sound.

Fortunately there are alternatives to creating positive thought that can yield similar results. For example decreasing the amount and intensity of negative thoughts by putting 120 bits of focused attention on your brain, as we discussed earlier. This is also easier than creating positive thoughts. When you stand on one leg, put one hand on your chest to monitor your breath and spell the word "elegance" backwards, you will be very hard pressed to create any thought beyond the one related to the activity. And the good news. Decreasing negative thought content is as health promoting as creating positive thoughts and carries less risk of negative interference as described earlier.

Data is also on your side. Studies show that optimism (which I take the liberty to compare to positive thinking) itself is not related to blood pressure overall. When optimists are in a bad mood, their blood pressure is just as high as anyone else's. It is the level of pessimism that is related to chronic blood pressure levels (Räikkönen et al., 1999). More recent data confirms that absence of pessimism is more strongly related to positive health outcomes than presence of optimism (Scheier et al., 2021). I hope you accept that optimism is an expression of positive thought and pessimism is an expression of negative thought.

Perhaps without realizing it, while reading this book, you have already practiced thought-alteration skills. Many of the exercises you've encountered so far engage you in focus that limits the brain's ability to create negative thoughts. At the beginning of this chapter, I made you imagine the word "joyful." I purposely picked an emotion that I knew has a reasonable chance of not making you feel worse.

Let's take this a step further. Write the word "joyful" in the air virtually. Literally move your hand when you air-write the word. Always take a breath in between letters. This exercise has an even higher chance at decreasing negative thought content. There is a good chance you can actually not think at all because your 120 bits per second of brain capacity are engaged on writing imaginary words in the air.

I claimed earlier that when we change our mood and our physical state, our thoughts will obediently follow into healthier territory. By writing imaginary words in the air about desirable emotions, there is a good chance you will decrease negative thought content and shift the body towards feeling better, often closer to the emotion you have been writing in the air.

Try it out for yourself. Pick an emotion that you would like to experience and write it in the air while you are breathing. Which emotion did you pick? What are you discovering about yourself?

DEFAULT NETWORK

As we are discussing the various components of thinking, how to take advantage of them, and not fall victim to their hidden pits, there is another piece of information I want you to understand about your brain, so you can either adjust to its evolutionary flaws or challenge yourself to change. As researchers increasingly have the technical ability to look at what happens in the brain when we think, they can apparently differentiate different brain states. One state is generated by what is called the cognitive control network, which is activated when we focus on a particular task. We have discussed how we can utilize our ability to activate focus, so let's look at another network that researchers have named the default mode network, which as the name implies is activated in the state the brain "defaults" to when it is not engaged in an externally oriented, goal-oriented task (Andrews-Hanna, 2012).

The default network processes information regarding the self, such as memories of events and facts about one's self or reflection about one's own emotional state. But it also thinks about others. Thinking about what others might or might not think and what their thoughts could mean. The network is also responsible for social and moral evaluation. And it loves to remember the past and think about the future.

Unfortunately it is often up to no good in a state of distress. It tends to comment on what we should or shouldn't do, it time travels either to the past or the future, and it constantly makes references to what we think about others and what others think about us. Remember this happens without any input from the outside. The brain self generates the thoughts. Sounds pretty exhausting to me.

The default mode is not per se a bad thing. On the contrary, if we are balanced and in a good mood, we can pleasantly daydream and think about a solid sense of ourselves and what geniuses we think we are today. Unlike focused attention, the default network is stimulus-independent and task-unrelated mind wandering. With emotional difficulty, however, and as you have learned cancer constitutes an emotional challenge, this default mode network can be taxing. It turns into a self-deprecating rattle. Instead of turning inward for reflection, we brood on abstract problems or fixate on obstacles to solving concrete problems (Zhou et al., 2020).

The exercises in this book take advantage of the fact that there exists a separation in the kind of task the different networks perform. Instead of letting the brain blabber on, some of the exercises force the brain to switch into a focused state.

Going forward I suggest that you occasionally check in with your thoughts and decide if you are engaged in specific focus mode or in default mode. If your thoughts are in negative default mode, I suggest you switch to a focused task. Once again I suggest this based firmly on my observations that it is easier to shift your focus than to successfully disengage from negative banter. As I discussed in the context of thought seizures and metacognition, to stop thought at will is often not that easy, but to focus on a particular task, like knitting or counting backwards by subtracting sevens from 100, has a greater chance of getting you out of the default mode.

There are other advantages to focusing on a particular task. I have observed clinically that the more specific and structured a focus is, the less likely you will have interference from unwanted thoughts and emotion. Less control over the cognitive content carries a higher chance of experiencing surprises. Instead use the network that is wired for focused cognitive tasks, which in my experience carries a smaller risk of interference.

When you walk yourself through the alphabet, alternatively thinking of words in two languages or count backwards while focusing on breathing, you are not just taking advantage of the brain's limited ability to process a lot of information simultaneously, you also utilize a network that will result in more relaxation overall. I don't know if physiologically this corresponds to shifting out of the default network, but it seems to work.

ATTENTION RESTORATION THEORY

While the ability to shift focus helps you not to stay in the negatively blabbering default network, let's be clear that focusing on a task is still effort. In order to not exhaust your focusing network, you might want to give it a little break on occasion, particularly with an option that takes NO WORK on your part! There are ways to make the brain do the work for us.

Yes, we can force our brain to do something beneficial without having to work hard at counting or imagining words. I love this because it adds ease to your life rather than making you work hard at tasks, even if they make you feel well. The fancy word for this process is called Attention Restoration Theory (ART). According to ART, interacting with environments such as nature will invoke parts of the brain that allow the parts that are responsible for focused attention a chance to restore (Kaplan & Berman, 2010). When we're out in nature, the brain does not exhaust itself with a directed attention-solving task, such as how to not get run over by a car or with having to make complex choices about how to treat your cancer most effectively. The attention is captured by features of nature itself, which does not pose the same challenge for the brain as crossing the street while someone honks at you. You do not have to do anything actively to watch a sunset. The brain will do it on its own.

Interestingly, when people interact with natural environments, they then perform better on tasks that depend on directed attention. Which means taking a walk in the woods or staring at nature images will not just make you feel better but make you think better. This is even true if you are prompted prior to your walk to think about something negative (Berman et al., 2012).

Marc Berman, the head of the Environmental Neuroscience Lab at the University of Chicago and a researcher on Attention Restoration Theory, also points out that you need to pick activities that constitute what he calls *soft fascination* rather than *hard fascination*. For example, if after an exhausting day at work you listen to soft music and let your eyes rest on the flame of a candle or a painting, your brain is more likely to recover than it would from watching a football game, bingeing on an exciting Netflix show, or getting lost in YouTube. The latter activities involve competition, possibly violence, or scenes of betrayal, all of which can tap into your own unresolved problems, creating "a kind of internal noise that would lead to excessive demands on direct attention" (Kaplan & Berman, 2010). As a cancer patient, you must allow your brain to restore itself, to get some rest from all the challenging experiences, traumatic interactions, and important decision-making.

The brain only constitutes 2 percent of our body weight, but it uses 20 to 25 percent of our daily energy. And if you always have the same part run in overdrive within the wide electronic networks, it will wear itself out.

Take a moment right now and assess whether you are thinking about the past or the future. Also, take a moment to reflect on whether you are benefitting from wherever your thoughts are. Are you benefitting from mulling over millions of times the same question of whether your presumably poor nutrition or lack of exercise or the stress at work caused your cancer? You will never get an answer to this question, and you will likely strain your brain. If you relate to what I just said, let your eyes rest on nature or a picture of nature or let your eyes search the sky for a bird.

BE CURIOUS ABOUT YOUR THOUGHTS

While I proposed various options how to deal with thoughts, shift away, or alter them, it's important that you not outright reject them. Even if they seem "negative," they might carry information you can learn from as we discussed earlier in the section on **Thoughts Are Stand-ins for Needs**. Remember that thoughts can represent needs. Since you are learning tools to avoid being overtaken by your thoughts, you might have more bandwidth to use them to your advantage.

Take the sentence "I am worried it is just in my head," which is a sentence I hear from patients frequently. This thought implies that "there is something wrong with me" and that you judge certain thoughts (I often have to slap my wrist to refrain from saying, "Yes, it is in your head because that is where thoughts reside." But I don't. That would add insult to injury). But rather than just dismiss the thought, I learn from your revelation that you hold self-judgment. The expression of the thought gives you and me important information. If you realize that you are judgmental towards yourself, you open the door to directing your thinking toward a different, more desired place of acceptance or curiosity or whatever characteristic you want to develop.

I hope you can see that I am trying to coax you in the direction of observation, analysis, and understanding of your thought experience rather than engaging in negative judgment about your thoughts. This approach increases the probability of effectively changing an experience over the usual approach of categorization and judgment.

I want to remind you that thoughts are a window into your inner, mostly unconscious experience. They are extremely valuable, even when they feel unpleasant. As I have illustrated with the unwelcome thoughts about the funeral arrangements, thoughts can guide us to what we need. We get to poke our nose into our personal Pensieve.

You will often hear me recommend going *with* what is, not against what is. Whatever is, is. I agree with T.S. Eliot that "Humankind cannot bear much reality," but I also believe that it is beneficial to get closer to our reality. We have to operate within the bounds of the brain's physiology.

The process of unearthing "reality" is a challenging part of my work. People often don't accept the laws of the mind. Not out of ill will but from inexperience and lack of understanding and fear. I encourage you to remove self-judgment about your thinking, behavior, and emotion, but acknowledge that it is not easy. We develop elaborate schemes to quiet the mind when we are overwhelmed by what it wants to tell us, and I understand that some realities are very painful to bear.

I vividly remember Pierre, who after a shoulder injury had a very difficult recovery, and the prolonged healing was baffling everybody. I will never be able to prove that there is an association, but I can't help speculating that his childhood reality, when his father used to pin him down and threaten to break his arm if he didn't behave, might have left a traumatic imprint that affected his recovery. Let's not blame our minds and bodies but instead have deep empathy for them if they don't want to remember certain realities.

So far we have seen that a lot of thoughts aren't accessible; they have a life of their own, and our processing speed is a little slow. But I hope you have also learned that with a little curiosity and tolerance you can use your thoughts, and if need be, change them. Let's explore further how to do that and not let monkey mind get the better of us.

THE ART OF CHANGING THOUGHTS

In the introductory chapter to this book, I mused what motivates us to change. Even if we are motivated to change, can we? The big questions are, can we effectively change thinking, and if so, how?

I picked the section on thoughts to discuss change in more depth as I find it one of the more challenging areas of change. But what I am about to say also applies to emotions and body sensations as I will discuss in those respective chapters. And I want to emphasize again that it's often easier to focus on a specific task or decrease negative thought content than it is to create a positive thought, or even more challenging, to replace a negative thought construct with a positive one.

If you believe "I will never succeed," it will be easier to diminish the brain's ability to create the thought that you won't succeed by doing a yoga tree pose (you'll hear the details about the physiology in **Chapter 6** on **Body**) than to alter your brain into establishing the neuronal network for believing that "I often am easily successful." But if you are set on positive thinking, I want you to remember that learning how to do it is the equivalent of learning another language, in part related to overcoming our negativity bias. And like learning a language, it requires learning one word and one phrase at a time.

I want to echo the TV news anchor Dan Harris, who in his book *10% Happier: How I Tamed the Voice In My Head, Reduced Stress Without losing My Edge, and Found Self-Help That Actually Works: A True Story* (what a title!), amusingly inspires you not to expect a change overnight but to gradually change yourself towards the better. Stay realistic, and do not expect the kind of overnight transformation offered by Byron Katie or Eckhart Tolle. While I believe that sudden transformations like the ones they describe can happen, I also believe that epiphanies like theirs usually do not commonly result in overnight change. While you may come to some profound insights, do not expect instant results; they're just not standard for normal (in the statistical sense of the word) people, particularly normal people with cancer.

The distress of cancer is so pronounced that expecting to go through the experience and come out of it suddenly enlightened and altered is terribly unrealistic and unhelpful for most. If it happens, great, but do not let your desire for change be an additional stressor to your already distressed cancer life. For most of us, change is gradual and comes with work.

I am happy about the things people experience in self-realization workshops, like the ones given by Tony Robbins. There can be moments of insight that feel exhilarating and life altering, such as the conviction never to commit the same mistake again. Moments of happiness when you feel connected to yourself. But this is what they are—moments. When you go back to chemotherapy the next day, you will be hard pressed to recreate the feeling you experienced at the life-altering weekend with guru X. The good thing about workshops like these is that they allow you to connect to yourself in a meaningful way, cognitively as well as emotionally, but they are neither instant fixes nor thought and feeling maintenance programs.

In the next chapter, which is all about emotion, you will read about the instability of emotion, a fact which is often a source of great disappointment for self-help workshop participants. After a rich and fulfilling experience, you expect to sustain the experience. That, however, is incompatible with the physiology of human thought, emotion, and body. Just going about your daily business, or worse, exposure to distressing events will be enough for you to revert to reactive patterns that were conditioned before.

To undo conditioned patterns, we have to gradually dismantle the neuronal network in the brain that represents them. This is why I say that thought patterns change gradually. At the end of my own workshops, I always caution participants that, as wonderful as it is to be part of a bubble in which they could learn and explore, they now have to carry the experience back to their lives to implement and consolidate—and that comes with work and time and patience and often many disappointments along the way.

EXERCISE TO CHANGE THOUGHTS

Now that I have asked you to be patient with your expectations in changing thoughts, I want to walk you through an exercise that I encourage you to use for future practice. If the practice at first sounds and feels weird, keep in mind that we have to accommodate that "the conscious mind allows itself to be trained like a parrot, but the unconscious does not," as Carl Gustav Jung taught us earlier. Here we go.

I'm using the belief "I will never succeed" as an illustration, but you would be using the sentence that expresses whatever thought you would like to change.

Start by taking a breath and saying out loud, "I will never succeed" followed by another breath. Observe your physical and emotional response after saying it and breathing. You might feel tension or sadness, or you might relax or feel a sense of relief. Just observe whatever you feel. Then take a deep breath again and say, "I wonder who I would be if I occasionally believed that I could succeed sometimes." As before observe your feelings, thoughts, and sensations that are associated with saying the sentence. I hope you will feel a little physical or emotional opening, a sense of wonder, a body shift that allows the brain to consider a change of unconscious belief.

You can do this exercise with any kind of sentence. If you're someone who is afraid of recurrence, your sentence would be, "the cancer will come back." After a deep breath, you say the sentence, take a breath again, and follow it with saying, "I wonder who I would be if I occasionally believed that the cancer won't come back." If this sounds scary to say out loud, you can start with a more innocuous belief.

SPEAKING CANCER

Earlier in the book, I mused about what makes us change. Let me say again that sudden change can happen, but more commonly people grow gradually. I was inspired by the eloquent description of the process in Dan Harris' book. In my own work, I use metaphors to show patients how to make gradual change. If a patient asks how to "quiet the mean bully in my head," I might talk about the similar process of learning a language. We cannot learn a language overnight.

If you went to China without an interpreter or a dictionary, communication would feel scary. Telling yourself that you should be fluent in Mandarin will not help you, but learning one phrase at a time will make your next trip more pleasant. Learning "cancer language" without a bully in your head is no different. As I have already mentioned, my patients often have a sense of heightened urgency in the face of—sometimes real, sometimes presumed—death. Many cancer patients do not die from cancer, but it often feels to them as if they certainly will and soon.

If you want to consolidate your practice, and figuratively speaking "learn Mandarin," you can use the bullying sentence. Take a breath, say, "I have a mean bully in my head," followed by a breath and the second sentence, "I wonder who I would be if I occasionally quieted the mean bully in my head?"

It is intriguing that the mind generates these strange thoughts, and I have mused about their possible purpose. With the same sense of urgency that patients want to pack all unlived opportunities into a presumably shortened life, they want to speak "Cancer" overnight. It is not realistic. It often adds distress rather than relieve it. Anyone who has mastered the overnight "cancer skill," please contact me. I want to be your devoted student.

Only very few of us have the luxury, devotion, or privilege to dedicate our lives to meditation; most of us cannot even afford a workshop or visit a spa. We have to get through life, and sometimes we have to go through life with cancer. Let's grow and heal with realistic expectations.

CHANGING THOUGHT THROUGH BODY

Sometimes thoughts don't fire rapidly like a machine gun or blabber in the default network. Thoughts, like emotions, can ebb and flow and very much depend on our mood and our physical state. Have you ever noticed how your thoughts can totally differ depending on how you feel emotionally and physically? At night thoughts can often take on an overly worried, even paranoid flavor. In the stillness of the night, there are fewer alternative activities, and thoughts are a convenient, albeit often unpleasant, activity filler. Nothing else to fill the 120 bits per second!

As we've seen, thoughts are also not always based in the reality of the situation. At night, in the void of other activity, you may absolutely "know" that you will fail the entry exam to whatever or be absolutely convinced that your boss thinks poorly of you. During the day, the exact same exam might seem conquerable, even an engaging challenge, and your boss might appear to be very manageable. Same exam, same boss, but depending on your state of mind, the assessment of it is altered.

I want you to pause and reread what I just said. Humans spend a lot of time reasoning that it is unreasonable to think you will fail the exam and thus you should not think it. I consider that a waste of your time. Better to change your mood and your physical state and watch as your thoughts obediently follow into healthier territory. That is in part why exercise works. It is not just about the endorphins flooding through your body. Keeping the body engaged leaves less capacity for the brain to think crap. It is worth not taking thoughts so seriously, unless the thoughts genuinely help us solve problems effectively and efficiently. Even the most recent set of exercises have a physical component to them without you setting foot on a treadmill. Breathing moves the chest and calms the nervous system, and that helps facilitate changing your mindset.

Even though you might think that I have painted a doomsday picture of the brain's ability for thought, I want to remind you that you *can* change. We are going to take advantage of the fact that the brain is quite a vast storage container, with retrievable information outside of our awareness, built like a patchwork computer with limited processing speed and unpredictable retrievability. We have discussed many aspects of cognition and thought and how you can use this knowledge to promote health without stepping into thought traps. I hope I have given you tools to have more control over what is going on in your head and tools not to allow unhelpful thoughts to create havoc in your body. Now let us turn to emotions.

CHAPTER 5.

Emotions

The same way thoughts can get hijacked, so can emotions. No one knows this better than cancer patients. You are standing in the grocery checkout line, exhausted after a grueling course of radiation, trying to juggle picking up your children from daycare with buying basic ingredients for the yet-to-be-cooked healthy meal when you, to your own dismay, burst into tears. How embarrassing! The cashier might look away or mumble a feeble sorry while the person checking out behind you gets annoyed, or meaning well, puts their hands on your shoulder and you dissolve even further.

Or maybe you think of yourself as an exuberant and positive person and feel completely discombobulated when you find yourself erupting into an irritable and grouchy tirade every time someone asks you a question. You might even be realizing for the first time that you *have* emotions.

Sounds familiar? Just as your thoughts seem to have a life of their own, so can your emotions.

A considerable proportion of my patients are scared of emotions. They don't want to connect to them but at the same time are concerned that not expressing them might make their cancer progress or return. Tricky catch-22! But just because the shock of cancer jolts you into a different universe—one that often is filled with different or new, more intense or more frequent, and at times even out of control emotions—does not mean you have to retreat from them. What I want you to know is that the same way you can affect your thoughts to better suit your purposes and goals, so can you learn not just to manage your emotions better but to actually take advantage of them or change and shift them if you do not like them.

DEFINITION OF EMOTION

Before we return to cancer-specific components of emotions and how to change them, I want to make sure we have a common understanding of what constitutes an emotion. Many of us have a sense of what an emotion is but can't produce a definition when probed. I stated in the beginning of the book that I use Google definitions, not because they accurately define but because Google searches have become a standard source of knowledge, forcing me to at least confront the content. Google defines *emotion* as a "strong feeling deriving from one's circumstances, mood, or relationships with others" and an "instinctive or intuitive feeling as distinguished from reasoning or knowledge."

Therein lies the first problem. These definitions casually throw around words like "feelings" and "mood," along with emotion. Have you ever considered the difference between emotion and feeling? And how much do you even need to know about the physiology of emotions and how they differ from feeling or mood in order to feel at ease with them and take advantage of them?

From Google we learned that emotion is an experience that is different from thought and somehow related to your surroundings, including people, which I find interesting. It makes it sound as if an emotion cannot happen autonomously. What do the experts say? Lisa Feldman Barrett, in her book *How Emotions Are Made*, which I mentioned earlier, emphasizes the individuality of emotions. She offers the most detailed account I have come across of the individuality of how emotions are made and their purpose, pointing out that "an emotion is not a thing but a category of instances, and any emotion category has tremendous variety."

Let's look more closely at *categories of instances* and start with experiencing them!

THE EXPERIENCE OF EMOTION

You might think you know what emotions are, but let's do an exercise to see if that is true. Take a moment and state a few emotions. First state the emotion you are experiencing right now, then the strongest emotion you felt today, and then dig for the most pleasant emotion of last week, and last but not least, identify the emotion you experience most frequently on any given day.

Always take a breath in between explorations.

Could you easily connect to and define your emotions? If you struggled, you can go back to Figure 4 in the **Introduction** for guidance.

This exercise does not come easily to everybody. People will say things like, "I don't like my teacher, my boss is a jerk, or my partner has abandoned me." While you can probably sense the emotion behind the words, these are not in fact examples of emotions. They are thoughts and experiences associated with emotions. In these examples, the emotion itself is probably something close to a mix of anger, frustration, or disappointment.

THE PURPOSE OF EMOTION

The reason I encourage people to develop the ability to identify emotions has to do with their usefulness. As I briefly discussed in **Chapter 2** on **Advocating for Purity** emotions (like thoughts and body sensations) are a detection and signaling system for internal processes. They also give us hints about external processes, such as an unsupportive boss or an insane health insurance system. This internal barometer system has proven useful as part of human evolution. In times of danger, our ancestors needed a way of alerting themselves to run away from the tiger that appeared from behind the bush. Emotions serve as an alert signal to jump into action.

I have already pointed out in **Chapter 3** on **How We Process Events** that scientists have argued over whether we run away from the tiger *before* we develop fear or if emotion and behavior happen concurrently. My personal system clearly cannot distinguish their apartness, even if science is going to prove that there is one.

What about you? Do you sense something and reflexively jump into (unfortunately often quite thoughtlessly) immediate action to the dismay of your loved ones? Or do you perceive an emotion and deliberately evaluate the emotion before you take action?

Scientists also argue over the extent to which emotions arise from the brain or the autonomic nervous system, the latter about which you will learn in depth in the coming chapter on **Body**. From a practical perspective, what matters is that you have emotions. When searching to describe your emotion and you want to keep it simple, pick from angry, happy, sad, or fearful or simply note, "I experience something."

I will be discussing the physiology of emotions shortly, but if you don't care for evolution, anatomical details, and brain circuitry, you can skip those sections, but you do need to know some fundamentals if you don't want your emotions to trip you up during the process of dealing with cancer. As I mentioned already, emotions are highly individual, but unfortunately they are also unstable and not super predictable when the system is under duress.

INDIVIDUAL DIFFERENCES

Understanding individuality of emotions is essential for cancer patients. I explained earlier that everything exists on a continuum and that the statement is true for emotions as well. As a reminder, continuum means that within humans there is a broad range of experiences and that everybody is included on the spectrum of experiences, as far-ranging as they might be. Remember what Lisa Feldman Barrett showed us in *How Emotions Are Made*: people differ greatly with respect to intensity and expression of emotions and feelings.

Experiences can range from "I don't feel any" to "I drown in them." Some people do not have easy access to their emotions or don't express them. In order to navigate your own emotions, it is also important to realize that how you experience emotions might be quite different from how the person you interact with experiences emotions and feelings.

As a society, we still carry a legacy from earlier times when any expression of emotion was considered improper. In fact many people still have difficulty accessing or expressing their emotions and have to learn how to do it. Lately the pendulum seems to have swung the other way, and we are encouraged to express our emotions. Ideally I want you to allow them to ebb and flow naturally.

Again what's important to note here is that the quality and quantity of emotions individuals experience can vary widely. What evokes my sadness and what my sadness feels like might not be what makes you sad or how you feel sadness.

Though we still see remnants of emotion suppression, excessive expression is not unheard of either. I have worked with people who attend workshops specifically developed for the expression and cultivation of emotion. Let me say this: While it is admirable working on becoming emotionally literate, if you still feel bad after years of expressive emotion and crying sessions, you might want to consider a different approach.

I believe, as with many things, that moderation is most conducive to health. And more importantly, that we ought to connect to what feels most natural to us. Just because someone tells you that you should either suppress or express emotion does not mean they're right. You have to know what's right *for you* and go from there. Remember the word "should" as a signal that you're dealing with a likely obstacle and recalling the inspiration from early in the book: "I promise myself that I will never use the word 'should' again." It is a good practice to not just wean from the word but also the pressure of the actions that are attached to it.

STABILITY AND CONTINUITY OF EMOTION

Another common misconception about emotions is that they are stable. In fact we tend to expect positive emotions to be stable but then dread the stability of negative emotions (which I believe is one of the reasons patients often do not want to engage with their emotions at all). When you feel good, you want the feeling to hang around, but when you feel shitty, you want that feeling to go away! But neither of these is a reasonable expectation. Emotions fluctuate.

Emma Seppälä, Science Director of the Center for Compassion and Altruism Research at Stanford University and author of *The Happiness Track*, describes emotion as an ebb and flow, a description I used earlier for thoughts. They both come and go. One second we feel something, and the next we might feel something else. If we can accept that emotions are fleeting, we need to address the fact that people seem to desire to sustain what they consider positive emotions, such as happiness, while they hate to get stuck in what they consider negative emotion, such as resentment or anger. We cannot sustain good emotions, but we can facilitate reconnecting to them when we feel something we don't enjoy. That's the good news. You can learn to shift your emotions.

Patients will sometimes tell me, "I don't do sadness." Well don't worry, sadness will do you! It is physiologically impossible to sustain any single emotion. Instability is their basic nature. You can take specific steps to bring on the emotions you desire, as you already explored when I had you imagine the word "joyful" and will further explore with exercises in this chapter. We can also practice the Buddhist idea of emotion neutrality. If I understand correctly, they do not differentiate "positive" from "negative" emotions. If we can simply experience emotion from one second to the next and know that they fluctuate, we liberate ourselves from wanting (or expecting) to experience continuity of "good" emotions.

EMOTIONS UNDER DURESS

But it's not just individual differences and fluctuations of emotions that are important. As a cancer patient, you can greatly reduce your distress by understanding how emotions change under extreme stress. The same way thoughts can get weird with distress, so can emotions. As mentioned in **Chapter 4** in the section **Thoughts Under Duress**, the stressful force of cancer constitutes duress. The body confuses the threat, "cancer," with a lion and reacts accordingly. You revert to how an animal would behave when wounded. Roar, run away, or play dead. You are in survival mode, and basic emotions can become more prominent in survival mode. After an exercise section, we'll distinguish between more basic or primary emotions and more sophisticated or secondary ones in the section about the **Physiology of Emotion**, but for the purpose of cancer, let's look at the primary ones, which are crucial to understand.

As you know from your own experience, cancer patients often feel a heightened sense of urgency and intensity. Emotions feel raw and sometimes unfamiliar. Everything starts to feel "primary," which I associate with "primal." Stripped to its essence. Everything becomes about survival, and getting someone to take care of those dirty dishes in the sink can feel as urgent and upsetting as reading the latest research article about your condition.

I had already discussed in **Chapter 4** on **Thinking** in the section on **Memory** how cancer can constitute trauma, but it is not just the imprint we have to pay attention to. Emotions don't only become more primal under duress, they affect the ability of the emotional brain and the rational (or thinking brain) to communicate with each other. When we feel distress, the communication between the two functions of the brain can break down, and the emotional brain takes over. Earlier I quoted Bessel van der Kolk, who notes that the rational brain is basically unable to talk the emotional brain out of its own reality. You might experience a strong feeling, and even though your brain generates the concurrent thought that you don't want to feel the feeling, you will feel it anyway. No matter how much your rational brain tries to tell your emotional brain to stop feeling that way, the emotional brain will overrule the rational.

What I want you to take home from all this is: Don't be surprised by strong emotions and don't be surprised by unsuccessful attempts at reasoning; and get used to behaving like a wounded animal. That does not mean you have to remain a wounded animal. Read on to see how but not before doing another exercise first.

MORE EXERCISES

Let's continue on with one you already started in the section on The **Experience of Emotion**. Take a moment to assess your emotions. Not to judge them or yourself but just to identify them. Always take a breath in between assessments.

What are you feeling right now?

Are you struggling to identify emotions, or do you know right away what you feel?

Take a breath.

Are you reflecting to determine your emotion, or are you sensing something in your body to make the assessment?

Take a breath.

When in doubt, you can always resort to core emotions: happy, sad, fearful, and angry, or an approximation of one of these.

Take a breath.

Take moments in between your observations to also focus on breathing in and slowly breathing out.

This idea here is to find your personal place on the broad spectrum of human emotionality. Do you have access to your emotions? Do you enjoy feeling them? Do you want to express them? Who are you when it comes to emotion? This exercise is not intended to produce feeling pleasant or energized. It is simply an assessment of what takes place inside. Identification of what *is* increases the probability of being able to change it.

PHYSIOLOGY OF EMOTION

While it is perfectly okay to stay with exploring emotions as an alert and barometer system, some patients find it helpful to go deeper. I got myself into a bit of trouble about this once when, while teaching a workshop, I suggested that we keep things *simple*. A workshop participant felt deprived of the richness of exploring her emotions. Point well taken and a good reminder that we must honor our individual differences. What is right for the goose is not always right for the gander! And so I will delve deeper for the ones of you who find it helpful.

Let's use fear as an illustration. Remember when I introduced Mr. Baldwin at the beginning of the book and used the example of a car driving at you? Most of us know what it feels like to experience that kind of fear. Again the scientific debate over whether the ability to jump out of the way to avoid getting run over precedes the feeling of fear does not matter for practical purposes. It happens very fast, and we can thank evolution for that. Otherwise the streets would be littered with human pancakes. Jumping out of the way is an adaptive survival mechanism that we have developed over millions of years to enable instantaneous assessments about our surroundings and respond with appropriate behavior.

The conventional view has it that our basic emotions are generated by an evolutionarily older part of the brain called the limbic system. You might also hear that this view has been challenged, and researchers now suggest that the activity of the brain happens through a system of networks rather than in specific anatomical locations (LeDoux, 2016). I find the term "basic" or "primary" useful. The basic emotions are the ones that are most closely linked to body responses. The close association to body reactions is reflected in our language. "Tremble with fear" or "shake with anger" is something you easily can experience as a cancer patient.

There is even some debate in scientific circles about which emotions are basic emotions, but all agree that "anger, happiness, sadness, and fear" form the basic set. Paul Ekman, an emotion researcher, has proposed along with others that "surprise" and "disgust" belong in the set of basic emotions as well (Ekman, 1992), but his view has been challenged. If you read *How Emotions Are Made*, you get yet a different perspective. Feldman Barrett argues that emotions are a highly individual experience based on a complex blend of evolution, experience, and adaptation. But the most important message from her book is that your emotions are yours and only yours and are often not comparable to the ones had by your next-door neighbor, or anybody else for that matter.

I hope I haven't gone too far down this rabbit hole of scientific debate. The different opinions are not really relevant for you personally but mainly offer you a glimpse into how researchers think about—and still don't fully understand—daily experiences you probably spend little time thinking about yourself. Having this basic sense of how science looks at emotion might help you not get lost in the jargon if you delve more deeply into the science literature. What is most important is that you have a concept that there is an experience called emotion and that the experience can be useful, or if you don't pay attention, can drive you bananas. More fundamental still: there are emotions, and you will experience them, like it or not.

Susan David, a Harvard Medical School psychologist and the author of the book *Emotional Agility*, also suggests that we not avoid emotions. She advocates that in order to experience emotional agility, you first have to "show up" to your emotions and face them, whatever they might be. She believes that showing up is an important prerequisite that allows you to more easily "step out" of emotions and not be consumed by them.

Remember in the previous chapter when I likened speaking "Cancer" to speaking Mandarin? Speaking "Emotion" is similar. You can start with identifying core emotions the same way you would start accumulating the basic vocabulary of a foreign language. From the core set, you can expand slowly, particularly if you are new to the process of identifying emotions. If you love more subtlety and complexity, there are dozens of emotions you can explore. If it is pleasurable for you, by all means revel in them. But please do not worry. Detailed dissection of your emotions is not a requirement for successfully focusing on your health and dealing with your illness.

Figure 7 helps you play with identifying emotions if you want to go beyond the core few. What I like about this way of categorizing emotions is that it takes the intensity into account and organizes the emotion along two axes, from pleasant to unpleasant and from mild to intense.

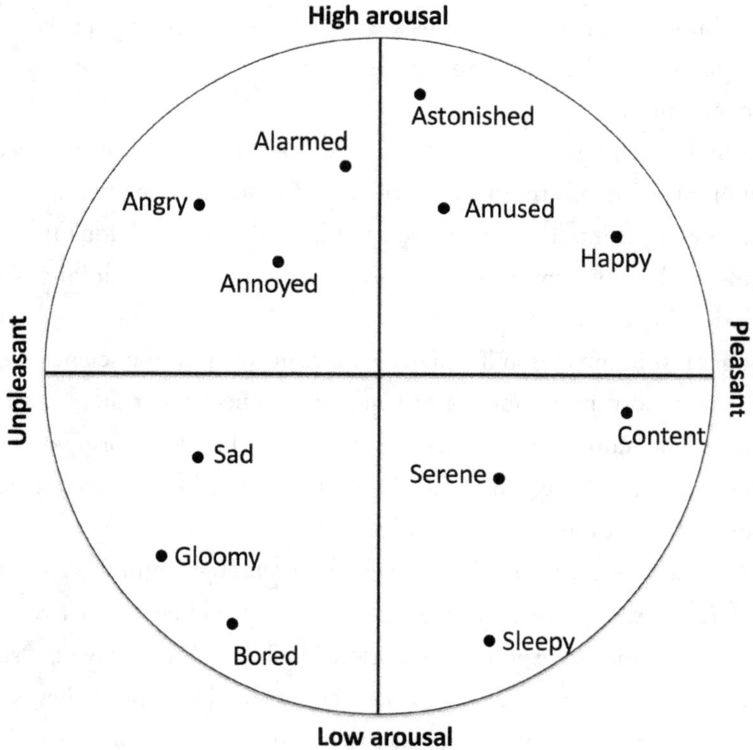

On the horizontal line (or axis) is what is sometimes described as the valence of an emotion, another way of saying "pleasant" or "unpleasant." The vertical axis expresses the intensity of your emotions, which is also called arousal. The lower left quadrant shows low intensity, unpleasant emotions; the lower right quadrant lists low intensity, pleasant emotions, the upper right quadrant lists high intensity, pleasant emotions, and last but not least, the upper left quadrant lists high intensity, unpleasant emotions. I find this map helpful to orient myself in identifying my emotions.

Compare for example happy and content. They both are pleasant, but happy has more energy to it than content, which feels a little calmer. Angry compared with sad. Neither of them feel very good, but anger has clearly more energy to it than sadness.

An additional differentiation is to minimize the risk of projection. Marshall Rosenberg, a psychologist, and author of the book *Nonviolent Communication*, whose work grew from the tradition surrounding Carl Rodgers, discourages the use of loaded words like "abandoned, ignored, pressured, threatened, rejected, betrayed" to describe your emotions because these words judge (Rosenberg, 2005). They imply a victim and a victimizer. In **Chapter 8** on **The Concept of Human Needs,** you will practice how to keep your list of emotions clean of projection and how this approach improves your health and effectiveness and minimizes that you misattribute your experiences to an external cause or person.

Ideally we could learn from our Buddhist friends who, as I mentioned earlier, do not differentiate "positive" from "negative" emotions. I am very much on board with that idea, but the Western view of dichotomizing emotions is so ingrained in our society that it will remain a model in this book, thus my elaborations on positivity and negativity of thoughts and otherwise.

SECONDARY EMOTIONS

While primary emotion often has a physical component as we just discussed, more complex or secondary emotions are more closely linked to parts of the brain that are evolutionarily newer (give or take a few million years) and often involve some thinking and self-reflection. You have just heard me state that you can keep analysis of emotions simple unless you enjoy reveling in detail, but I want to expand on that statement. I believe that as a cancer patient, you can benefit from educating yourself about secondary emotions because understanding decreases the risk of distress when your own or others' emotion flare. I ask you to bear with me here if the details seem laborious to follow.

Because of their different wiring and purpose, primary and secondary emotions are not very coordinated when you are under siege from cancer distress. As I have mentioned, cancer can catapult you into intense emotions that can be fast and furious. The wounded animal brain is on display! Since the secondary emotions often involve thinking and self-reflection, these thought-flavored emotions convolute the picture.

Research informs us that the electrical pathways for basic and secondary emotions are different and that even within basic emotions, there are circuitry differences (Zhang et al., 2019). Neuroscientist probably wouldn't be happy with my simplification, but I interpret the literature to mean there is some seriously complicated stuff going on in our emotional brains. Primary emotions that are evolutionarily older are processed by different fibers than secondary, more complex emotions, which the brain evolved more slowly over time, when we gradually moved from the jungle to our presumably more sophisticated form of living.

Remember the section in **Chapter 4** on **Thinking** that described how the development of the brain follows the patchwork laws of building and remodeling a house? The process gradually evolves and does not always produce a perfectly designed and functional house. Same is true for emotions. Researchers argue about the specifics, but I want you to understand that the wounded animal part is responsible for how your emotions often play out when distressed by cancer.

Basic emotions are processed very fast (your heart beats immediately when the car cuts in front of you) compared to the subtle exploration of "Do I really love Mary?" which involves slower circuitry and more thinking. Reflect on this for a moment. Do you find this difference to be true for yourself? Do you experience the flushes of anger, the chest pressure of fear, and the tears of sadness? When you assess whether you feel "content" versus "satisfied," does the evaluation become a little brainier and explorative? "Content" and "satisfied" will give you a physical sense of ease but not the raw directness you feel with primary emotions.

Figure 8 returns us to the core principle of this book. It repeats Figure 5 but adds emotions into the picture. I placed basic emotions below the yellow box to align them with body since the two are so closely associated. I placed secondary emotions above to align them with their "brainier" association with thought and reflection.

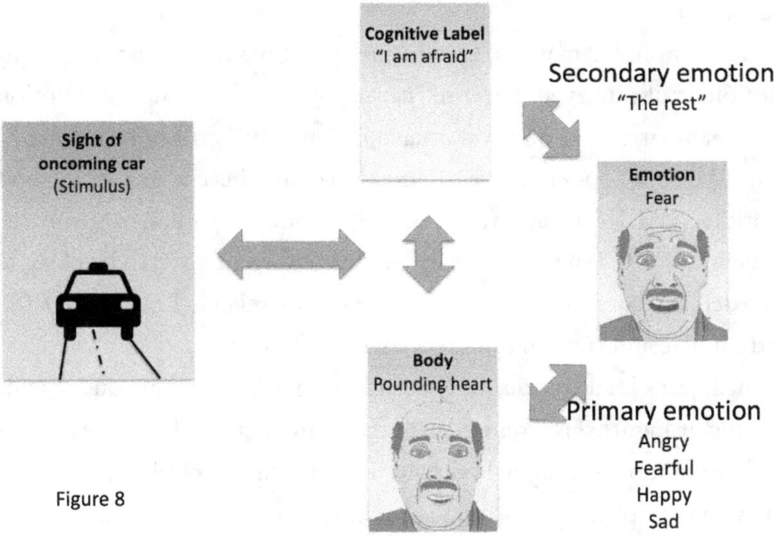

Figure 8

EMOTIONS UNDER DURESS 2.0

I know that it can be mind-bending to learn about the physiology of emotions, but I want you to have an understanding not just so you can see how your emotions can get hijacked in the face of cancer but to show you how emotions often lose their sophistication and are more "basic" when confronted with the stressful experience cancer. When you turn on survival mode (or rather your body turns it on for you), your "secondary" emotions lose their sophistication and go "primary" as we discussed in the section **Emotions Under Duress**. As I mentioned before, the body confuses the threat "cancer" with a lion and acts accordingly. The body (and the human that is sitting in it) runs away or plays dead at a time when it needs to be at its best to make effective decisions with respect to treatment and other important aspects of cancer circumstances. Instead you spend your time in the grocery line disintegrating or yelling at your partner or experience some other personal version of being emotionally hijacked. It is this disconnect, this sudden irritability and hair-trigger reactivity, that makes it important for you to understand emotions, so you can avoid becoming their slave and can instead be at your best emotionally and cognitively to solve your problems.

To complicate matters, it's not just the illness itself that can trigger an emotional tailspin; even the word "cancer" can evoke an intense emotional response similar to the one you'd have if you had a grizzly bear in the living room. We have pondered several times how thoughts can impact the body and emotions, and I cannot stress this point enough. Joseph LeDoux, the researcher at NYU I mentioned earlier, states it succinctly, "To feel fear, all that is needed is a cognitive belief that you are in danger" (LeDoux, 2020). That pretty much sums up the experience with cancer.

Being sick is automatically associated with believing that you are in danger. Looking at Figure 8 is a reminder of the grim likelihood of entering a vicious cycle of emotions-thought-body discomfort, unless you develop the tools to deal with your physiology. And I am reiterating that the vicious cycle can spin in both directions. Emotions have an impact on thoughts and body as much as the other way around.

While it is good and healthy to have emotions and to have changing emotions, being constantly scared is not beneficial because it can elevate your heart rate and keep your body in a constant state of distress. This is a worry I often hear from patients. "I cannot be stressed because stress is not good for me." It is true. Actually it is only somewhat true, and I will elaborate on stress versus distress in the next chapter when we discuss the body in more detail. But it is true that some forms of stress are not good for you. The distinction matters because it can help you minimize the "distress about distress" many cancer patients feel. For now let your brain register the fact that emotions are an important part of your physiology, they are not related to being weak, and they function as an important information system for our being.

TIME TO GET CURIOUS ABOUT EMOTIONS

The same way I advocated being curious about thoughts, I also advocate being curious about emotions. Mark Wolynn, a psychologist in Northern California, and the author of the book *It Did Not Start with You,"* states that "when we try to resist feeling something painful, we often protract the very pain we are trying to avoid." Emma Seppälä writes in her book, *The Happiness Track*, that "we know intuitively the powerful impact emotions have on us." I would generally subscribe to both of these ideas but only after a careful assessment of personal differences. I think emotions are worth exploring, not just because they function as such a good signaling system but also because they so easily mess with your well-being if you do not pay attention, even if you are someone who does not have easy access to your emotions.

Having said this, however, my primary interest here is in helping you find your place on the spectrum of emotional experiences. Some people are expressive about feelings, some people less so or not at all. Some people have strong feelings, for some the emotional experience is subtle. Some people become emotionally more expressive under duress, others wall off their emotions. Whatever it is for you personally is what you will have to work with. So it is worth to know who you are emotionally.

To translate these ideas into daily life, however, is not an easy sell to many patients, and a few obstacles need to be removed first. As I already mentioned in the introduction to this chapter, a considerable proportion of patients are caught in a catch-22: on one hand, being scared of emotions and not wanting to connect to them. And on the other hand, feeling concern that if they don't express them, it might make their cancer progress or return.

But the difficulty goes beyond ambiguity about emotions. We also have preconceived notions about emotions. "I should not feel this way," is one of the most frequently heard sentences in my office. Many of us were not allowed a natural approach to letting our emotions happen when they arise but were taught ideas about them, unfortunately often not always fruitful ones.

"Emotions represent weakness," is a popular conditioned thought, and we tend to have distress or self-judgment-evoking associated thoughts with emotions. And as I mentioned in the section on **Metacognition** in the previous chapter on **Thinking**, this tendency for self-judgment is an obstacle to really understanding what's happening inside of you and do the best with what you have or improve it. Furthermore experiencing emotions for many of us feels like losing control, not an appealing process, particularly as it resembles the experience with cancer which in itself is often perceived with an associated sense of loss of control, instability, unpleasant surprises, and uncertainty. Patients question how adding the unpredictability of emotion benefits them. Who wants to feel anything, particularly if negative beliefs are attached to the experience?

A core part of my work involves easing patients into recognizing the value of emotions as a valuable source of information. Teaching you that you will feel a certain way, even if you decided that "you should not," convincing you that you will feel something even if you don't want to and helping you remove your conditioned ideas about emotions open avenues of discovery, expansion, and to the surprise of many, welcomed control. As a cancer patient, your orientation towards emotions matters particularly as your emotional experience often changes with cancer. For some of you, this might mean becoming more emotional or more expressive, for others it might mean becoming less emotional or less expressive. If you understand who you are with respect to emotions, you will be less unsettled by their changes and have more influence over how to change them to your liking.

Most of my patients start to buy the idea that emotions can be helpful when I point it out—and promise that experiencing emotions will not kill you. If you argue back that Debbie Reynolds died from the strong emotions elicited by hearing about her daughter Carrie Fisher's death, I will point out that it was not the emotion sadness that killed her but a very complex physiological cascade that indeed can get triggered upon a traumatic and shocking event, which is poignantly called broken heart syndrome. It is like knowing what is under the hood of the car. It will eventually save you a few trips to the shop. Let's not just investigate what's under your hood but change a few screws yourself.

MORE EXERCISES

The purpose of the first two rounds of exercises in this chapter was to explore what you experience when you try to access the emotion currently present rather than attempting to produce a chosen one. Again, by identifying what the emotion is, you increase the probability of changing it. Now let's see how you do with producing an emotion and not just identifying one.

You can also try to remember what you saw in Figure 7. Identify the quadrant of intensity and valance if you can't precisely name your emotion. You can peek at Figure 7 to help you make the assessment. You can also pick an emotion from Figure 7 or simply decide what it is you would like to feel right now. For example, take the emotion "pleasant." Close your eyes and imagine the word "pleasant" in front of your mental eye. If you have difficulty visualizing, you can simply write the word in the air as if you were writing on an imaginary blackboard.

Imagine the letter P or write the letter P virtually by moving your hand in the air and then take a slow breath, focusing on slowing and extending the exhale. Then turn your attention to the letter L. Gradually walk yourself through the word by focusing on every consecutive letter while taking a breath in between every letter.

Once you have spelled out the whole word, with breaths between each letter, briefly check in with yourself to determine whether or not you notice the desired shift. Do you feel "pleasant?" Don't be disappointed if you don't, as it takes some practice. Remember we are learning the alphabet and vocabulary, so we can become fluent in a foreign language. We are not there yet. You will evolve and become more proficient as you keep doing these exercises.

And if you can create an emotion with this exercise, you can also change it by picking another emotion you would like to experience, air-writing it, or imagining it in front of your mental eye. Your body automatically retrieves previous associations, and because of the close association between cognition and emotion, you have a good chance at experiencing the imagined emotion in the process. The same way there is the art of changing thought, there is an art of changing emotion. But be thoughtful what you wish for. This process also works for emotions that you might not want to experience like anger or resentment.

By now you are an emotion expert, so to close this out, let's look at some other issues and options that arise with emotions.

DISTINGUISHING BETWEEN EMOTIONS AND FEELINGS

People tend to use the words *emotions* and *feelings* interchangeably. For the purpose of getting you through cancer in one piece (literally speaking), it does not matter what you call it. We are talking about an inner sense, sometimes soft, sometimes alarming, that calls us to pay attention. If making distinctions between emotions and feelings doesn't interest you right now, by all means skip to the next section, **Emotion-Associated Actions**. If you're game, read on about my attempt at distinction.

USC neuroscientist Antonio Damasio devotes a whole chapter of his book, *Descartes' Error*, to the difference between emotion and feeling. Let's look at what "feelings" are with an intriguing example. There is a smart emeritus psychologist at the University of Washington in Seattle named John Gottman. Early in his career, Gottman noticed that he had a knack for working with couples. Over time he developed a keen sense about which of the couples he worked with would eventually divorce. His level of accuracy in predicting which marriages would survive and which would not was an eerie, uncanny 90 percent. Curious about what he perceived, he started to design studies to help shed light on possible explanations. He "felt" something that needed further exploration. What he felt was not a simple emotion like fear or happiness.

Remember David Eagleman's book, *Incognito*, discussed earlier? We sometimes "feel" something, we sense something, but we can't define it. It is not a basic emotion like "angry" or "sad" but something more complex. The experience of "feeling," writes Damasio in *Descartes' Error*, is "tuned by experience, when subtler shades of cognitive state are connected to subtler variations of emotional body state."

Gottman and his research partner started looking for the patterns of interactions between spouses that Gottman might have been "feeling" during his work with them. After much work, he discovered that one of the kisses of death for marriages that were doomed to fail was a feeling of "contempt" for the partner. Contempt is a more elaborate experience than anger. The point I am trying to make is to stay curious about your emotions and feelings and what they represent as they add clarity to help change and take action.

By no means do I want to confuse you with nomenclature. We can settle on calling it emotion or feeling and leave examining the difference to the scientists. Joseph LeDoux, the NYU researcher we met earlier, sheds light on the confusion when he states that "the common English use of the term emotion is at best a poor notion, for emotion is a rich and complex theoretical concept with many subtle aspects" (LeDoux, 2000). There we go.

EMOTION-ASSOCIATED ACTIONS

An additional challenge is how wounded animals behave, particularly wounded human animals. In the previous chapter on thinking, I discussed thoughts and actions and how difficult it can be not to impulsively act on thoughts. There is an analogy with emotions. Thought-associated actions can pose problems but so can emotion-associated actions. We have seen that emotions are alerts to act for the evolutionary purpose of survival. When life is or feels threatening, our survival mechanisms kick in. What makes this tricky is that some of these responses (emotional or otherwise) are not adaptive but in fact maladaptive to the circumstances. The action we feel impelled to take is in fact unwise.

This disjointedness we experience might be an evolutionary stage. Maybe one day the more primitive parts will modify or die off in response to the fact that our lives are not under threat nearly as often as they were when danger lurked everywhere. But for now, part of our brain follows the laws of an earlier stage of our evolution and other parts follow the laws of newer evolutionary stages, and they are not always well-coordinated, particularly when we are distressed or traumatized.

Bessel Van der Kolk makes an analogy to a smoke detector. We want the smoke detector to alert us to a potential fire, but it will also go off with a smoky oven. Once we hear the alarm of the smoke detector, we make an assessment of the actual danger. When we are distressed, we tend to misinterpret the cause of the alarm and have a diminished ability to differentiate between different levels of danger. Everything feels like a burning house, even if we are just dealing with burnt cookies in the oven. You need to call 911 for the first but not the latter. The analogy for you might be to getting multiple MRIs for a headache because in distress, a tension headache can eerily and easily feel like a brain tumor.

There is another way that emotion-associated actions can get us in trouble. Remember how Daniel Levitin compared the development of the brain to building and remodeling a home? We develop elaborate schemes to quiet the mind if we are overwhelmed by what it wants to tell us. I believe that to be true for emotions as well. I see this commonly, not just in patients with cancer. We try to quiet our emotions by taking certain actions. How often do you snack, have a drink, run an errand, redecorate the kitchen, or smoke a cigarette to avoid experiencing an emotion? Are you familiar with the restless feeling that makes you walk to the refrigerator or reach for the candy jar?

Next time your body walks to the liquor cabinet, even though you swore not to let it, see what happens if you first sit on the sofa for five minutes and try to identify if you have an emotion and tolerate it if you detect one. It won't be fun, but you might discover that the emotion disappears or changes—without the drink or candy bar. If the experiment becomes too unpleasant, you can still grab a candy bar five minutes later to get the relief. The behavior is maladaptive but provides relief nevertheless until you get the courage to do the experiment another time. There are any number of books out there to help curb behavior detrimental to your health. Unfortunately we are often unsuccessful, and our coping strategies come with considerable collateral damage because we don't recognize that eating the cookie or drinking the beer is an attempt at alleviating emotions and distress.

If you are told to engage in healthy behavior and you want to engage in healthy behavior but then engage in unhealthy behavior instead, you will feel worse than before! What I suggest is that you try engaging in some of the exercises from this book before reaching for the drink, the snack, the cigarette. Let the exercise soothe the emotions. Then see if you still have the urge to engage in the unhealthy behavior.

Sometimes, however, the opposite can be true. Not taking action can also be motivated by fear, and that can also be detrimental. Often the non-action serves to protect you, but sometimes you pay a price for non-action as well.

Maybe you can find inspiration to act despite fear, as James Neil Hollingworth who wrote under the penname Ambrose Redmoon expressed so succinctly, "Courage is not the absence of fear, but rather the judgment that something else is more important than one's fear."

So it goes both ways: when you're feeling an emotion, you can explore if the action you feel urged to take is a way to not feel an emotion that might be worth feeling, or the emotion you feel prevents you from acting in ways that would be beneficial for you.

EMOTION-ASSOCIATED THOUGHTS

Remember when I called emotions and thoughts twins joined at the hip? We have already learned that thoughts evoke emotions and emotions affect thought. Let's revisit this connection again from the perspective of emotions. In the last exercise, I took advantage of the connection. The same way I leveraged the processing capacity of the conscious mind at 120 bits per second to teach you how to NOT think something (see **Chapter 4**), we can use this phenomenon to produce an emotion.

When I asked you to imagine or air-write the word "pleasant," I took advantage of all kinds of brain circuits that have been previously established and activated that have a good chance at producing a pleasant emotion. While you imagine the word "pleasant," your body automatically retrieves previous associations, and because of the close association between cognition and emotion, you have a good chance at experiencing the emotion "pleasant" in the process. Like all exercises, this will not work for everybody as not everybody has the same visualization and associative capacity, but if it works for you, please use it.

The same way we can use cognition to help create pleasant emotions, it unfortunately also works the other way, as many of you experience frequently. The thought, regrettably common in cancer circles, "I need to express emotions so I do not get cancer" can be a constant evoker of fear. "I cannot express emotions because they are a sign of weakness" is another classic mentioned earlier. Imagine the internal mayhem that occurs when these two conflicting sentences coexist.

In the previous chapter, we established that thoughts can evoke emotions. What I'm asking you to do now is separate emotions from associated thoughts. Associated thoughts are not per se bad. They can be a useful source of information. They might reveal conflicting needs or unrealized desires. And once you have identified that the underlying needs are conflicting, you have more options for change. Or you can challenge the acquired belief that emotions constitute weakness and eliminate the internal conflict. Your body will reward you with a sigh of relief. You will create a physical sense of ease.

This cognitive-emotional coordination—bringing curiosity to what your mind is doing and teasing apart the emotion from the thought—is one of the harder parts of my work but also among the most rewarding. Once you realize and get proficient in this process of self-regulation, it becomes very liberating taking charge of your inner processes and provides a sense of manageability. Self-regulation goes beyond thinking and emotions. Self-regulation is the ability to adaptively regulate your attention, emotions, cognition, and behavior to respond effectively to internal and external demands.

TEARS ARE YOUR ALLIES

Before we turn to the next chapter on **Body**, I want to discuss one physical aspect of emotion: tears. I briefly touched on tears in the context of emotions. Tears come often with the experience of cancer. When you experience emotions, you might also experience water flowing out of your eyes. People call it crying. I call it water out of the eyes. Even though the water is strictly speaking a body production, I have placed this section into the chapter on emotion because most people experience that emotion-body collaboration as mostly emotional. I hope to change that. The same way I have advocated that emotions be viewed as body products (and remember that the brain is part of the body), so are the tears that are produced with the emotions. Unfortunately people generally are not very gracious towards emotions or tears.

The book *Crying* by Tom Lutz describes the historical background of how tears and emotions became stigmatized and were associated with weakness. I am glad to find that I am not the only one that calls this a cultural error with monumentally negative impacts for society. To teach children that tears and the emotions associated with them are a sign of weakness and should be suppressed would be like telling people to stop peeing. You can hold it in to some degree, but sooner or later it will flow (literally speaking).

Holding in or suppressing emotions has an accumulative effect that is physically exhausting (which is my equivalent to what Wolynn said, "When we try to resist feeling something painful, we often protract the very pain we are trying to avoid").

Since everything in the body is in a continuous ebb and flow, you'll find that emotions release quickly when you allow them to. People often feel relief after releasing emotions and tears, particularly if they overcome their association with "weakness."

I have been criticized for my desire for depth. If you want depth on tears, read Tom Lutz's book. Three hundred and fifty-two pages devoted to crying? Now that is what I call thorough! Here is the gist: CRYING DOES NOT CONSTITUTE WEAKNESS. Crying can be very good for you! Particularly in the presence of someone telling you that everything will be okay and not to cry.

If water wants to flow, let it flow! Crying is a parasympathetic activity. You are about to read what parasympathetic means, but as a rule of thumb, the more parasympathetic, the merrier.

I hope I have made a pitch for the importance of emotions and how to use them. Now let's move to the third entity in Mr. Baldwin's ping-pong, the body.

CHAPTER 6.

Body

Let's get something out of the way right up front. Despite its title, in this chapter, we will not be discussing everything about the body because not all parts are equally relevant to your well-being as a cancer patient or to your understanding as a person involved with cancer. I will devote more attention to those parts that are most easily and quickly influenced. For example, you can immediately and palpably influence your heart by simply altering your breath. Influencing your liver, however, is a more elaborate process involving monitoring certain behaviors, such as the amount of alcohol you drink or what you eat or don't eat or what medication you take and how they interact with each other. The liver is as important to your overall health as the heart, but you will hear less about it in this chapter because I want you to focus on the things that will bring you rapid relief.

When it comes to dealing with the distress of cancer, some parts of your body are also more involved than others. What you will hear most about in this chapter are how the brain and the nervous system can get adversely activated in cancer patients and what you can effectively do about it. But because the brain and nervous system are intimately linked to all the other organs in the body, I still find it helpful to consider the body as a whole. Thus this chapter on body.

To understand the entity *body* better, remember first that the body is made of cells. Cells stuck together like little Lego bricks. Some cells help produce thought, other cells help us pee or cry or digest food. You'll remember preamble one in the beginning of the book in which I pronounced that we are a heap of cells. A reasonably designed and coordinated heap of cells but after all just a heap of cells.

Even to speak of body separately from thought and emotion is tricky, since thought and emotion are body, aka cell, productions. Strictly speaking all cells are "body" cells. I didn't realize it until I put the polishing touches on the final edits of the book that I put the chapters in order of thought, emotion, and body, claiming at the beginning of **Chapter 4** on **Thinking** that the order was arbitrary, but now I am not so sure. I suspect my unconscious bias went along with the prioritization of putting thought first, and it is probably also not a coincidence that the chapter on thought is the longest. Even though I think of myself as balancing body and brain, I am probably more cognicentric than I fully realize. But as I evolve as a physician and healing guide and also in the process of writing this book, the importance of body has been climbing up the ladder in terms of relevance and usefulness as an interventive practical tool.

As I pointed out earlier, some people make a distinction between body and brain. Lisa Feldman Barrett separates the two in her book, *How Emotions Are Made*. But in this book, when I use the word "body," I mean the totality of you, every cell, including your brain cells. Again the nomenclature is not the point. What matters is that you have an understanding that emotions and thoughts have something to do with brain cells.

There is a certain irony in the fact that I managed to trichotomize Mr. Baldwin into thought, emotion, and body, as if I support Descartes' view of their separation. Even with my great efforts to change the way you view thought and emotion as body products no different from others like sneezing, crying, or peeing, I am stuck trying to integrate an old but very ingrained dogma with modern brain science. Since humans tend to be thought—or even more generally cognition—heavy, I often find that people have little awareness of the "non-thought" parts of the body.

I was struck by what I read in the obituary of Kenneth Baker, the long-time art critic of the *San Francisco Chronicle*, in which his wife was quoted as saying that, for her husband, Aikido was a critical path to counteract "the somatic numbness of daily life" (Winn, *San Francisco Chronicle*, October 13, 2021). This lack of experience and understanding about our somatic existence comes with numerous disadvantages, which I expressed as point two in the preamble: "Misinformation about and misinterpretations of the function of cells have led to many misconceptions of human functioning, leading to unnecessary suffering."

I recommend that we understand cells, so we can take advantage of the knowledge of the functioning of cells to feel better (Point three in Preamble).

Let's first turn to the anatomy and physiology of the body parts that are important for cancer distress before we look at stress and distress and the difference in more detail. In the introduction, I made my case for moving away from the concept of psychopathology in association with cancer and focusing instead on distress. When you understand the physiology of distress, many of your current experiences will make more sense. My hope is that understanding the physiology of distress will become a companion in your life the same way I hope the bald gentleman from Figure 5 has become an easily accessible fixture in your head.

THE BRAIN

One important system of cells in the process of cancer experience is the brain. Think of the brain as the head of a squid or a jellyfish. From the center, you have many tentacles that lead to the periphery, which would represent nerves (which we will discuss next). Some people like anatomy, some like imagery, some prefer abstraction. You can either go over pictures about the brain online or make up your own image. Important is that you have a sense that something is sitting inside your skull and that you can relate to it as an organ, the same way you can relate to your heart beating and your lungs breathing. That brain of yours is pretty much involved in anything you do. Familiarize yourself with it.

The "brain on a stick" image that I mentioned earlier symbolizes the human disconnect between our brainy existence and the rest of the body. When describing Descartes in Figure 2, I used an image that represented this "brain on a stick" quite well. But I want you not just to have an anatomical idea of the brain but a concept of its connectivity and circuitry. In your search about images of the brain, also look at images that depict the electronic network aspect of the brain.

As you learned in the chapters on thought and emotion, the brain can get flooded with thoughts and emotions. The brain gets overactive, which some of my patients describe as a brain "on fire." One patient shared a photo of a glass sculpture called "The Sun" by Dale Chihuly that is exhibited at the Salk Institute in La Jolla, California to illustrate what her brain feels like. It struck me how closely the photo of the sculpture resembles images representing the brain's networks. As many patients share, they experience a physical correlate or visual image or a temperature associated with their overactive brains. This can make imagery a helpful healing tool.

If you imagine your brain being visually "on fire" or feeling "too hot," developing an image of changing the color to something soothing or imagining a cooling sensation will often elicit a sense of relaxation, which is surely a desired goal.

THE NERVOUS SYSTEM

The brain is connected to the rest of the body through nerves. Nerves play a fundamental part in our ability to do a lot of things. Imagine wires coming out of a central computer and a switchboard directing action in the periphery of your body. These would be the arms of the squid I asked you to imagine earlier. Nerves are a good thing. You would not be able to walk, move your arms, write, go to the bathroom without them.

Many of the actions we take that are based on nerve activation are conscious. Take a moment to observe how you lift your arm. You can command your arm to lift, but when you look at the activity "going to the bathroom," you might realize that it is not as clear cut. While most of you have perfect control over going to the bathroom, you don't have perfect control over NOT going to the bathroom. At some point your body will pee, whether or not you like it. Let's first turn to the nervous system, over which we have no or limited control. Given its autonomous functions, it is called autonomic nervous system or ANS.

Autonomic Nervous System

The ANS connects the brain to pretty much every cell in our bodies. As the word autonomic implies, the ANS is responsible for regulating the body's automated functions like digestion or breathing. Now when we look at going to the bathroom, a mix of voluntary and autonomic systems are involved. Breathing is similar. You have some control over breathing. But you also know what can happen when you hold your breath or avoid going to the bathroom for too long. You cannot hold it endlessly!

The autonomic nervous system is like a freeway system on which information from the brain travels to the body and conveys information to the rest of the body to get the job done with whatever needs to be done, like move, digest, or breathe. This freeway also allows information to travel back to the brain. The ability of the brain to perceive, process, and integrate the senses from within the body is called interoception. The brain doesn't just know to go to the bathroom. When the bladder gets full, it sends information to the brain and says, "Heh, I am about to burst, let me go pee."

That communication is pretty cool and coordinated but unfortunately when the interoceptive signals arrive in the brain, cancer patients tend to misinterpret these signals the same way they tend to misinterpret emotions and thoughts. All of a sudden the urge to go to the bathroom turns into stacked thoughts: "Didn't I go already three times today? Am I going more often now? Is my bladder cancer back?" And as you have learned earlier, thought stacking paired with doubt is quite stressful.

The autonomic nervous system connects every organ to the brain and conveys information from the brain to every organ. But it is not just involved in how you breathe and when your heart beats, it also contributes to immune regulation, endocrine function, and thermoregulation.

The details of the physiology and anatomy of the ANS go beyond the scope of this book, but trust me when I say that the ANS is one of the most important systems in the body. The dysregulation of the autonomic nervous system that is often happening in patients with cancer also affects many people without cancer with many challenging health consequences (Benarroch, 2020). This dysregulation of the ANS is unfortunately often incorrectly reduced to only mean "stress." It always makes me a little crazy when I hear someone say that "it is just stress." Nobody who has an understanding of what the nervous system does would ever say that. So when you hear that something is "just" stress, don't despair and simply read on.

The ANS is itself divided in two parts, the sympathetic part and the parasympathetic part. If you want an image consult a book or go online to get an idea of this division. The same way the brain is challenged when it deals with cancer, so is the autonomic nervous system. The anatomical details are not important; what is important is that these two systems, the sympathetic and parasympathetic, are supposed to balance each other. The sympathetic part is commonly known as fight-flight-freeze. When it is activated, it stimulates the heart and increases the number of heart beats per minute. It also induces the lung to breathe more. Its basic function is to prepare the body to fight or flee, or at times freeze or play dead. It readies you to deal with whatever danger the world presents to you. The parasympathetic nervous system is responsible for functions related to resting, restoring, and reproducing. If you search online, you will read that the parasympathetic system is responsible for the stimulation of "rest and digest" or "feed and breed." Use whatever terms you like, as long as you understand the basic idea.

Unfortunately the autonomic nervous system is not as balanced as we would like it to be, not just in cancer patients but particularly not in cancer patients. This imbalance is at the core of what patients experience as distress. The same way the brain can be overactive and produce troublesome thoughts as many of you have experienced, so can the autonomic nervous system. It's important here that you know the term "sympathetic hyperarousal." Just as Mr. Baldwin in Figure 5 has become your frequent companion to remind you how you play tennis with your surroundings, so will awareness that the sympathetic nervous system has trouble staying balanced with its twin, the parasympathetic nervous system.

Let me repeat the key points. An overactive sympathetic nervous system is called sympathetic hyperarousal. Many cancer patients experience sympathetic hyperarousal. Many symptoms you experience are often but unfortunately erroneously attributed to cancer. They are not. They are based on sympathetic hyperarousal, and that arousal is part of how interoceptive signals from the body, aka symptoms, get misattributed to cancer. This is what Linda Carlson ultimately refers to when she reports that approximately 40 percent of cancer patients report significant distress (Carlson et al., 2012). Your brain and nervous system are overactive.

I am stressing this point (pun intended) about stress being associated with the ANS because most people view stress as something mental. While I see their point—as stress affects thought and emotion as I described in the two previous chapters—stress through activation of the nervous system is solely physical. It gets us back to the chicken-and-egg question about mind and body. Sympathetic hyperarousal is a physical event, a body event. This in itself ideally makes you feel better as you are less likely to misinterpret some of your symptoms. But if you don't want to go deep into understanding the physiology, simply follow the instructions for how to induce a parasympathetic tone on page 137 as you would follow a recipe in a cookbook. If you still wonder "what the bleep is ANS?" don't worry about it. By the end of the book, I'm guessing awareness of ANS will be your omnipresent companion.

Robert Sapolsky, a professor at Stanford University, wrote a wonderful book, *Why Zebras Don't Get Ulcers*, that describes autonomic function and dysfunction in helpful ways. For our purposes, Sapolsky's ideas about how our bodies deal with stress is instructive. There are different theories about stress and how stress affects humans. Sapolsky presents the "mismatch" theory. He suggests that as humans we still carry the version of the autonomic nervous system of our predecessors in the jungle, and as a result, cannot always differentiate between the danger level of a lion attack and the task of doing taxes. Both can result in a pounding heart, the strong urge to play dead (particularly in the case of doing taxes) or run away. Fear is the signal to the body to take action, and the autonomic nervous system coordinates this emotion-body interplay at light speed.

For the rest of the animal kingdom, the ANS still serves its original function, but humans can have a stress response in the absence of an actual stressor. Our ANS can be turned on when there is no real danger present. Thus the "mismatch" theory. This mismatch is common in cancer patients. You may be concerned that your cancer can recur or progress or that physical symptoms are cancer related, even when they are not. While this fear is at times based on an actual threat, it is often present even when you've been assured that your cancer is cured or the symptom is associated with an infection. The inability to differentiate between real threat and imagined threat adds considerable and unnecessary distress to your life.

I have used the lion analogy a few times now. It is useful once again. The body confuses the threat of cancer with a lion jumping at you from behind a bush and acts accordingly. You might flee (turn the other way when all it is is a well-meaning neighbor wanting to say hi), you might fight (fly all over the country to make sure you get the best treatment), or freeze (hide in bed when you are overwhelmed or lose your ability to think). With the awareness that your nervous system is simply making an attempt to adapt to what it (often erroneously) perceives of as a threat, you can make healthier adjustments. Your fight-flight-freeze mechanism gets tripped even when the threat is not real.

Start analyzing your behavior for fight-flight-freeze responses. Since being diagnosed with cancer, have you changed in ways that can be categorized in terms of fight, flight, or freeze? The following table gives you examples, and you can analyze your personal behavior changes since you were diagnosed.

Table 1

Fight	Flight	Freeze
Argue more	Don't answer the phone	Can't follow doctor's explana-tions
Snap at people	Isolate yourself	

As you can see, I advocate for understanding the autonomic nervous system, but if that is too arduous, just try the parasympathetic exercises. They will help you enhance parasympathetic tone, and that's never a bad thing. Many people in our society are sympathetically overactivated, even when they don't have cancer. Feeling relaxed is always preferable to feeling negatively stressed.

The interaction and relationship between the brain (also called central nervous system or CNS) and ANS activity is close. Interventions aiming at ANS activity are fairly simple. Enhancing parasympathetic tone and decreasing sympathetic tone can help you feel more relaxed and energized, and you get a two for one. You don't just feel better, parasympathetic tone also enhances creativity and helps with thinking and emotions (Deepak, 2019).

Parasympathetic Exercises (to help balance the ANS)

In Table 2 below, I offer some easy ways for you to experience parasympathetic tone. While some might intuitively make sense, others might strike you as weird. Just choose the ones that appeal to you or are easy to integrate into your day. But by no means do them all or do the ones that you have an aversion to because you think you "should." And make sure to repeat the ones you find most helpful at decreasing or eliminating negative thought content. This is very important, as we saw in the section above on thought.

Breathing out slowly	Sleep
Cold water for 10 seconds	Tai chi
Singing	Gargling
Yoga	Coughing
Meditation	Acupuncture
Laughter	Chew gum
Prayer	Massage
Exercise	QiGong

Many, many cancer patients are especially concerned about stress because they've heard that "it makes them sick." I understand that concern. Yes, it is true that being constantly and chronically sympathetically activated can have many negative impacts on the body. It elevates blood pressure, does not let you sleep, causes immune problems, and on and on. For the purpose of you dealing with your cancer distress, that's enough information.

If you want more details, you can read Sapolsky's book. He writes so well and entertainingly that you should have no problem making your way through it, even if the science does get a little heavy. But again you don't have to. Whatever you do, try these exercises. Balancing the autonomic nervous system is never wrong—with one possible exception: if you encounter a lion downtown. But don't worry. Your body will reflexively go into sympathetic action. You cannot overtrain your parasympathetic system and lose the sympathetic. Ever! It's just not possible.

How best to stay in balance is a hot topic these days (in the Western world at least). Many people in our society have an overly active nervous system. They are irritable, exhausted, have difficulty finding restful sleep, and have difficulty staying balanced. We have known for many years that pushing ourselves to perform will yield results, but if you increase the push and the stress to a breaking point, your performance will actually suffer. If you think of balance as the balance between the parasympathetic and the sympathetic nervous systems, things get a little clearer. It is the Yin and Yang of the Western world.

In my experience, people tend not to be aware that they are chronically sympathetically overactivated. They might not notice that their muscles are tense, that they don't sleep well, or that they are irritable but still go about their daily business. It isn't until they go on vacation, totally removed from their circumstances, that they might notice a change. But even though they might sleep a whole lot better and feel more chill chilling on the beach, they rarely come to the conclusion that they should change their lifestyle after they return from vacation. They simply assume that their "regular life" is normal and how they feel on vacation is a rare luxury or privilege.

Does this sound like you?

In my opinion, these folks have it entirely backwards. It is our responsibility to keep our system balanced. You need to help coordinate your heap of cells. Earlier I compared our bodies to Lego. Let's try that again. Imagine you are a structure made of Lego. Every cell of your body is a piece of Lego (This, by the way, would involve trillions of pieces of Lego). When you create a structure from Lego, you have to build it in a way that sticks together, where the pieces fit and it does not disintegrate at the first little push. The body is no different.

Somatic Nervous System and Muscles

I have already described the autonomic nervous system as being like spaghetti coming out of the brain. The autonomic nervous system is part of what is called the peripheral nervous system or PNS. The name makes sense as these are the nerves that go from the brain to the periphery. There are other nerve fibers that have a more voluntary component, the somatic nervous system. Again it is not at all crucial that you know all these terms, only that you have an idea about the function of these nerves in your body. Even if the idea is not a perfectly accurate representation of reality. Remember Heisenberg from the introduction?

"We must remember that what we observe is not nature itself, but nature exposed to our methods of questioning"? This should help you create exercises that make sense to you and are related to what you experience in yourself. It might not be nature, but it is your nature!

Part of the PNS are nerve fibers that connect to muscles. As many readers will have experienced, muscle tension is common with distress. When distressed we pull up our shoulders, tense our neck, or tap our feet. Many people are not aware of their body enough to notice, but they will be able to start paying attention when it is pointed out to them. Your body is a perfect sensor of distress, and muscle tension is one of the body's signals to you to pay attention. Your body can act as a barometer to help you implement strategies to relax. Instead of thinking of what techniques to use, such as hypnosis or guided imagery (both useful by the way), I want you to think of what technique is best suited to address your specific experience of body, thought, or emotion. It does not matter what exercise you use. As long as you find one that helps you feel your body settle into the "plane of balance and relaxation," you are on the right track to improve your health. Observe, for example, what happens to your muscle tension when you spend just a minute focusing on breathing in and breathing out. If that works, it's the right exercise for you! If you paused reading "plane of balance and relaxation" and were wondering what settling into it means, the exercise ahead on page 142 will explain.

STRESS, DISTRESS, AND POSITIVE AND NEGATIVE STRESS

After looking at the anatomy and physiology of the brain and the nervous system that create the experience of what we call distress, I want to discuss some terminology before we move to other parts of the body.

We seem to have a natural understanding about stress the same way we assume we know what emotions are. But do we really? Most everybody uses the word *stress* casually and frequently, but it is in fact confusing, as the term can refer to something either good or bad. Stress is an umbrella term for an activation of the autonomic nervous system with secretion of specific transmitters and hormones. The word does not tell us anything about the acuity or chronicity, nothing about intensity or the source. The word *stress* can be used to describe a broad range of experiences—from the excitement of passing an exam to the challenge of writing a research grant to the ongoing battle with cancer. Most people, however, attribute something negative with it. Google defines *stress* as a "state of mental or emotional strain or tension resulting from adverse or very demanding circumstances." The definition does not leave us a "good" or "neutral" stress option. The definition in fact sounds like what I refer to as *distress* or what some people would call "bad" stress. I suggest using the term stress neutrally the way physicists and engineers do. In the strict sense, *stress* is the "force per unit area applied to a material."

Does that sentence remind you of something? It is Mr. Baldwin in action. We simply describe that there is an external event called stressor, aka force, that applies itself to the material called Mr. Baldwin. We are not judging whether the stressor is good or bad, and we're not judging whether or not Mr. Baldwin's reaction is good or bad. We are applying the laws of the physics of stress to our ping-pong approach of life.

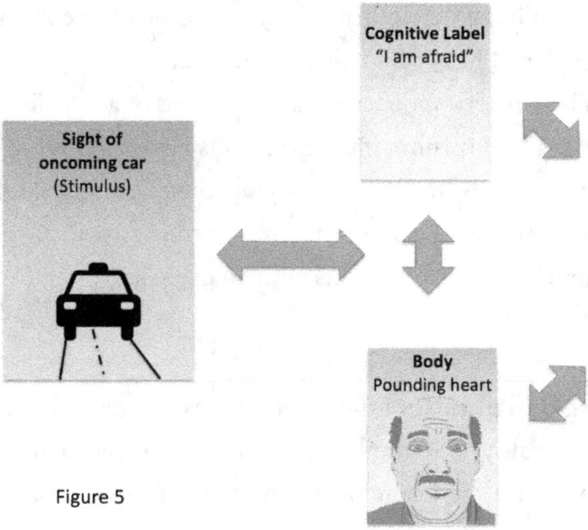

Figure 5

I encourage you not to use the terms *stress* and *distress* interchangeably but deliberately to differentiate if you are in the enjoyable state of positive activation or in the claws of distress.

Distress is the negative subcategory of the umbrella stress. The search engine mecca of Google defines *distress* as "extreme anxiety, sorrow, or pain." The choice of words in this definition is unfortunate. They are useless to helping you understand what happens to your body in distress. Let's craft a more helpful definition. Remember when I emphasized the importance of understanding distress at the beginning of the book? I quoted Linda Carlson, who states that distress is "not a precise clinical term." Did you notice that I never actually defined it? I simply relied on your incognito "knowing without knowing." Most of us have an understanding of what "distress" is when we use the word. In the context of cancer, let us settle that *distress* is *an unwelcome guest in our life creating havoc in the body*. Understanding the physiology of distress and its impact on you will help you deal with cancer-related distress.

From a cancer perspective, I furthermore want you to differentiate acute from chronic distress. It is not distress itself that creates havoc but the chronicity of it. Losing our temper once when the chemotherapy is not administered on time is one thing, but if the irritability that lies underneath is chronic, then you have to pay attention. That's why I always encourage you to do parasympathetic activities. They interrupt the cumulative process of acute distress piling on top of each other and turning into chronic distress. Your job is to give your body a break from distress by doing parasympathetic exercises. Once the distress of cancer has abated, you can resume the "normal stress" of job interviews and rock climbing. Let's practice this with an exercise.

EXERCISE

Imagine standing on a plane (not the one that flies) representing being in a state of balance, neutrality, and equilibrium. Imagine being in an elevated stage of activation by using the image of standing on a tree stump. Standing on top of the tree stump represents chronic activation of your nervous system. The higher the tree stump, the more activated you are. Most of us don't perceive that elevated energy state very well, but unfortunately it constitutes a health hazard. This chronically agitated state presents itself in subtle ways. Chronic irritability, disordered sleep, and low mood are examples you can perceive. Let's see if this exercise helps you to relax.

Take a breath with an emphasis on breathing out slowly and visualize standing on that tree stump. Let your body relax into the image, with your feet firmly planted on the stump. I asked you to imagine a plane, but maybe your fantasy has different plans. Look around to see if your imagination has placed you in a forest or a park rather than a plane. If your mind didn't present a natural environment to you spontaneously, see if you can produce an image of this tree stump standing in nature rather than be the sad remnant of urban redevelopment at a busy and loud intersection. Once you visualize your tree stump in nature, take another breath before you see yourself hop from one stump to another stump at a lower level, like a kid playing hopscotch, but with tree stumps. Take a breath every time you land on a lower-level stump. Eventually you will land in the plane of relaxation. Did the visualization and breathing help you come down from your elevated state of distress?

When I asked you to imagine planting your feet firmly on the tree stump, I had you engage with what is called kinesthetics, which refers to your awareness of the position and movement of your body, muscles, and joints. Engaging your body not just with exercise but awareness of balance and movement is a wonderful way of decreasing distress because it diminishes and sometimes even eliminates the ability to form thought. This is one of the reasons why yoga and tai chi are so parasympathetic. Focusing on your body definitely exceeds 120 bits per second processing speed and allow you to decrease thought content. This is a reminder of what I had mentioned in **Chapter 4** in the sections on **The Art of Changing Thought** and **Changing Thought Through Body**. By doing a yoga tree pose, it is easier to diminish the brain's ability to create the thought that you won't succeed, than to alter your brain into establishing the neuronal network for believing that you easily succeed by living with a mindset of failure. Or as I casually put it. Keeping the body engaged leaves less capacity for the brain to think crap.

Last but not least, I do have to mention "positive" stress. It's something you hear about, but I don't want you to get sidetracked by it. While I agree that stress can have good components, this rarely applies to cancer patients as the "positive" stress of taking on a challenge at work can't be compared with the distress of a cancer diagnosis. As a cancer patient, you would be doing quite enough to address your distress and its consequences on your body.

Kelly McGonigal, a lecturer at Stanford University, counters Robert Sapolsky's mismatch theory in her book *The Upside of Stress* and argues that we can't just transfer the fight-flight-freeze response from animals to people. In my clinical experience, the fight-flight-freeze response very much applies to people, particularly the ones with cancer! While a cancer diagnosis can lead to tremendous growth, I don't want you to add distress with the expectation that "cancer is the best thing that ever happened to me" as I occasionally have heard in my clinical practice. For most people, cancer sucks!

Stress is also not easy to study. Research on stress is often done in the setting of acute stress as chronic stress is difficult to study. Back in **Chapter 1**, we learned from Aaron Antonovsky that manageability, comprehensibility, and meaningfulness are factors that are helpful to focus on to promote health. On the other hand, there are factors that seem to increase the chance of a stress response.

Originally Hans Selye, who some call the grandfather of stress research, advanced the idea that any stressful situation can cause a stress response. However, a researcher in the 1960s by the name of John Mason modified that view (Lupien et al., 2007). In elegant research designs with novice and experienced parachuters, Manson could show that a stress response was most pronounced in situations of novelty, unpredictability, threat, and a sense of no control. Sounds familiar? He even termed a funny acronym. NUTS. This is what cancer is. It is nuts, literally and acronymically speaking. It is novel, it is unpredictable, it is threatening, and you lose your sense of control. Ergo, you will be stressed.

Ultimately we all experience distress in very individual ways and thinking of stress as "force (e.g., cancer, exam, divorce) per unit area applied to a material (me)" might be a good way to look at the impact our surroundings have on us and how we respond to them in the most neutral and personal way.

BREATHING—A BRAIN-NERVE-LUNG-HEART COORDINATOR

At the beginning of this chapter, I mentioned that I would not be covering all organs of the body, but the lung definitely gets a spot for its contribution to breathing. Breathing is one of the strongest natural inducers of parasympathetic tone—and it's entirely free! You have heard me encourage you several times throughout the book to focus on breathing, particularly on breathing out. And you probably noticed breathing is in the table on parasympathetic activities. Specifically breathing out with your lips pursed to create some resistance induces the parasympathetic nervous system. Bingo! Breath is also helpful to tickle the parasympathetic nervous system fibers that reside at the bottom of the lung.

This is what this emphasis on breath is all about when you are being sent to yoga, meditation, or breathing exercises. If you want to keep it simple, take deep and slow breaths to get the benefits of emotional regulation and well-being (Zaccaro et al., 2018). If you want to go into more depth, one of my very favorite books, *Breath* by science journalist James Nestor, is filled with suggestions and also explains the brain-nerve-lung-heart interaction quite well.

You have no doubt noticed that I always add a caveat for the people for whom breath does not come naturally or is even stressful. You just learned how important it is to balance your autonomic nervous system. To be in a chronic state of sympathetic hyperarousal is not healthy. To be in an ongoing fight, flight, or freeze state isn't healthy. This is where difficulty with breathing enters the picture.

When I first met Kay, an outgoing and goal-oriented VP of a Silicon Valley company, I wanted to help her relax with breathing. It wasn't meant to be. She hated it. Kay literally froze when I dared suggest that she take a deep breath. It took a few weeks for me to realize that suggesting she breathe was not just unhelpful to Kay, it was actually hurtful. It was traumatic. Only through gentle exploration, not unlike archaeological excavation of Pompeii, were we able to unearth several incidents in which Kay had frozen. Frozen as a way to stay invisible. "If I don't breathe, I will stay safe and protected" was, we discovered, her underlying motto.

Esther, a reflective, introspective, thoughtful young doctor also viewed my excitement for breath with skepticism, however, for a different reason. Breathing made her more aware of her body, which was physically uncomfortable given her ambiguous relationship with it.

When we associate *not* breathing with feeling safe, the suggestion of breathing with ease or deeply can feel unsafe. When not breathing allows us to protect against unpleasant body sensation, a suggestion of breathing can be experienced as uncomfortable. This is a situation in which the individualized approach I have emphasized throughout the book becomes fundamental on the path to success. This is individualized, targeted, precision medicine at its best.

If you happen to be in the category "breath stresses me out," pick other activities that are known to be parasympathetic from Table 2. Yes, ideally you want to focus on breathing when you sing, but give it a try. Singing is a nice way of sneaking in breath without you even realizing. Or forced laughter. You might ridiculously sound like a clucking hen, but try to have an open mind and give it a shot. If you feel self-conscious experimenting, watch people on

YouTube do it. What about gargling (preferably with ice water)? Definitely no breathing involved in that one.

If you think I'm making fun of you with these exercises (which I am definitely not, as there is solid science behind my suggestions), you can also engage with what is called exteroception, which relates to your interaction with external stimulation. I had pointed out earlier that some people are more visually oriented and others more auditorily. Now you can put the statement to the test. If you have internet access, search for binaural beats on YouTube and listen to some you like. Or if you want to explore your visual capacity, I have sprinkled exercises throughout the book that make you look at things, an example of visual stimulation. So even if breath is not exciting or even scary, there are many other exercises for you to do to facilitate a parasympathetic tone.

THE HEART

We've talked about the importance of the autonomic nervous system and how you can help yourself by inducing a parasympathetic tone. But there are a number of reasons why the heart gets its own section also. For starters you'll recall that early on I claimed without elaborating that distress can be identified simply by observing heart rate variations. Now is the time for the elaboration.

I'm sure you find it fairly easy to grasp that the brain sends signals to the heart to make it beat and contract (remember, it is a muscle), but I'm guessing it feels more unfamiliar to hear that the heart also talks to the brain. Yes, the communication is bilateral. There are "major pathways by which the heart communicates with the brain and body....Signals generated by the heart continually inform emotional experience and influence cognitive function" (McCraty et al., 2009). Yes, I did say earlier that when we experience an emotion, the heart is just along for the ride, but it turns out it's actually a bit more complex than that.

Most everybody is familiar with the idea that the heart beats at a certain rate and that you can feel that as a pulse on your wrist or neck. You can feel it as beating faster or slower. But there is another way to look at heart rate, namely by looking at the changes in the time interval between heartbeats. This is called heart rate variability (HRV). HRV is considered a measure that reflects heart-brain interaction and ANS dynamics (McCraty & Shaffer, 2015). The physiological details of neuro-cardiology (which is what this specialty area is called) are, yet again, not necessary for you to understand. The important message to take from this is that a) the heart is talking to the brain big time, and it's a good idea to listen, and b) the weird exercises I recommend here are all based firmly on the physics, chemistry, and physiology of the body.

If you're tired of all the exercises included here and want to use one of the many gadgets you can buy these days to promote your health, I recommend a heart rate variability-based biofeedback device. It is a nice way to help balance your emotions as well as your thinking, which as you read on, is an important thing to do.

AUTONOMIC NERVOUS SYSTEM, THOUGHT, AND EMOTION

I have already mentioned some of this in the respective chapters on thought and emotion, but I want to reiterate the deep impact your autonomic activation can have on your thoughts and emotions and vice versa. These connections cannot be emphasized enough.

Distress affects your thinking. You know that from personal experience. Now you can put it in the context that autonomic hyperactivity is implicated in poor decision-making in complex situations (Forte et al., 2019). This is something I see in patients with cancer all the time.

As patients experience fear, they are often overwhelmed with the complex decision-making they must do for their illness. They cannot process the information they hear from their doctor. That's why I champion reducing your sympathetic tone to be more relaxed during your doctor visit and therefore at your mental best. Sometimes people are so activated that they simply can't be fully present for their visits, which is why I also suggest always recording your doctor visits and listening to them later when you feel at more peace.

To study how distress affects thinking is challenging as no research design can mimic chronic stress perfectly (some researchers study women who take care of their disabled children as a stand-in model), and a lot of studies, as I mentioned earlier, focus on examining acute stress—like the one you would experience when you parachute out of a plane. But it is fair to say that distress affects cognitive functions, such as working memory, the mental workspace that underlies the control of thought and action, and cognitive flexibility (Shields et al., 2016).

ANS impact on emotions is not anything to take lightly either. It is hard to separate the body responses from the primary emotions since, as we've seen, they happen basically simultaneously. This instantaneous emotion-body action blend can be frightening to patients, as I described in the section on emotion. And remember it goes both ways. Emotions affect body, body affects emotion.

There is evidence to suggest that negative and positive emotions can be differentiated by ANS response (Cacioppo et al., 2000) and even that *specific* emotions, such as fear, happiness, sadness, and anger can be differentiated by ANS response (Collet et al., 1997, Kreibig, 2010). Researchers can hook you up to blood pressure monitors and pulse rate machines, measure electrical flow on your skin, and figure out that you are experiencing emotions in reaction to watching movies. It is not a perfect science, but we can now reasonably predict emotions based only on the readouts of the equipment measuring skin conductance and heart rate (Jang et al., 2019).

I say let's use this discovery to our advantage. You can alter your emotional response by altering your autonomic nervous system response. If you shift from sympathetic to parasympathetic state, your emotions will automatically shift, too. You cannot be angry while in a parasympathetic state. I emphasize this point to my patients. I explained the physiology earlier and gave you a list of parasympathetic activities to try; your thinking and your emotions will likely improve.

If you are marking up this book, get out your magic marker. Here goes:

IT IS EASIER TO CHANGE THE MIND THROUGH THE BODY THAN CHANGE THE MIND THROUGH THE MIND.

If I could pick just one health activity for my patients, I would pick to have them learn how to induce a parasympathetic tone.

CELLULAR HEALING

Remember our Lego analogy? We were reminded that we are composed of many, many (many!) cells. Now let's talk more about the biology of this cell composition. The significance that we are composed of cells dawned on me while reading Bruce Lipton's *Biology of Belief*, which I mentioned in the introduction. Bruce Lipton is a cell biologist. When culturing cells in petri dishes, he had already learned in graduate school to pay attention to the medium the cells were growing in. His description of how a cell thrives or shrivels depending on its milieu and what you feed it left a mark on me. When he provided healthy and nurturing conditions, his cells were happy and plump, but they faltered when the environment was suboptimal. And it made me think more about cellular healing and illness. Here's the thing. If you are made of so many cells, even when you have cancer, it is only a minority of your cells that are diseased. Not all of your cells are diseased. Even those aggressively reproducing cells that seem to get the upper hand over everything are still in the minority. Many cancer patients find relief in this fact. The majority of your cells are healthy. And you want to tend to those healthy cells as much as you want to get rid of the sick ones.

It might come as a little bit of a shocker that half of the cells in your body (that you want to keep happy) are not even human but bacteria. That's right. And many of those bacteria reside in the gut. I did not want to devote a whole chapter to the gut, but since it talks to the brain the same way that the heart and lung talk with the brain, I did want to mention the connection. As we are talking and thinking about cells and you are getting rid of sick cells with your treatment while keeping the healthy ones happy, the detour is hopefully worth a moment of your time. It is as important that we listen to the gut as the heart, even if what (or who?) is talking when the gut speaks to the brain is not always human! You want to treat your insides with respect. They are closely linked to the brain's well-being.

I encourage you to reflect on cellular healing and use guided imagery for that purpose. While you are working on eliminating cells you don't want—the cancer-mutated cells— you want to make sure that you don't forget to treat the cells that you do want very well. Send some gratitude and energy to the cells that are working hard to stay healthy for you. This idea links back to salutogenesis. Promote health!

If you are interested in reading more about cellular healing, I also recommend checking out *Cell-Level Healing* by Joyce Whiteley Hawkes. Professor

Hawkes was passionate about science and finished a PhD in biophysics at Pennsylvania State University in 1971. She did conventional research with sophisticated technology-examining cells. Her life took a very different turn when she had a near death experience after being hit by a glass panel while cleaning her house. She began to explore indigenous healing techniques and started to study spirituality and the connection between the body and emotions, and as she says, "discovered that emotional, mental, and spiritual feelings can have a profound impact on our bodies at the cellular level."

What fascinated me about the book was her ability to shift with seeming ease between her conventional world as a researcher and the world of spirituality. She will switch from pondering what mitochondria (the energy-producing part of cells) might need for optimal energy production to the vision she had of her mother and grandmother while knocked unconscious after her accident all in the same sentence!

Of course she is not the only one who had a fundamental shift in perspective after a near death experience. There is an entire body of literature on the subject. Since I did not have a glass panel shatter on me, I can't comment on what a near death experience feels like, but I can easily relate to the thought of reaching the body on a cellular level. Cells are little entities with electrical potential and follow the laws of electricity the same way a battery does. So when you hear the word *Energy Medicine*, it does not originate from some voodoo spirits but from the simple laws of electrophysiology of cells and cell structures.

ENERGY MEDICINE

Many methods in medicine are based on energy. Acupuncture and Qigong are examples. I've already established that we humans follow the laws of electrical current. Our trillions of cells constantly generate electrical activity to assist our cell metabolism and communication between cells, which then creates internal magnetic fields. It is no wonder that a whole branch of science studies how our electromagnetic body interacts with the external magnetic fields of our surroundings. So if you hear the term *Energy Medicine*, don't dismiss it. It is about electricity and magnetism the same way you can read in the physics book. It's not "woo woo" nonsense (though my physicist cousin disagrees with me).

I find it helpful for my patients to focus on energy. The same way I want you to look at energy the way physics defines it, I also want you to look at energy in the colloquial sense of the word, as in "I don't have any energy today." Many, many cancer patients struggle with low energy. They describe dragging, feeling fatigued, and not being able to get themselves to do anything. It can easily get confused with feeling depressed, but it is not. It simply reflects that the body's light switch has been turned off. In order to turn it back on (or at least get it to dim lighting), I'd like to remind you of something I mentioned in **Chapter 5** on **Emotion** and was illustrated with Figure 7. Feelings can be looked at from a quality perspective (pleasant versus unpleasant), as well as a perspective of activation (mild versus intense). Patients find it helpful to pursue activation. When you feel energized, feeling better and having more pleasant emotions often automatically follow. Instead of rigidly working on a better mood (of course you can do that also if it comes with ease), I have patients pursue energy and a better mood buddies along. You catch two birds with one stone.

Now that we've talked about the way we think, the way we feel, and the way our body works specifically in Chapters 4, 5, and 6, I want us to put all the cells back together in one piece. I called it **Thought-Body-Emotion: A Love-Jealousy Triangle** in **Chapter 2**. Let's move on to make sure that there will be more love than jealousy among the three.

CHAPTER 7.

Putting Us Back Together: We Are ONE (Heap of UNIQUE Cells)

By now I probably have worn out my welcome in all the back and forth about whether to separate thoughts, emotions, and body or consider them one heap of cells. What is it now: together or separate, separate or together? As usual the devil is in the details. It really depends on the purpose of looking at yourself. Different times and purposes call for different approaches. When everything feels like a blur of "incognito" disturbance, it can help to separate them. You pick a subset of a problem with the purpose to break it down into more manageable units. Improving the subset will improve the whole. We just need to remember that the subset is part of a bigger theme, the same way a puzzle is made of pieces. Without all the connecting pieces, the puzzle is not complete.

When you are haunted that you "should" be able to change your thinking, then read the chapter on thinking. You might find a morsel of info that helps with that. It will help convince you that you cannot just change your thinking because you think you "should."

If you want better access to your emotions, you might find exercises that allow you to do that. Or you might discover that being the way you are is just fine for what you need with your battle with cancer. The bottom line is we do what is helpful and furthers our cause.

Placing the discussion on positive psychology in this chapter illustrates my dilemma about the separate-versus-together question. What ultimately amounts to the same thing, being ONE, is best understood by looking at it from different angles.

POSITIVE PSYCHOLOGY

For a very, very long time, Western medicine focused on fixing illness rather than maintaining health and preventing illness. I am happy to witness during my lifetime the trend toward paying at least as much attention to wellness and illness prevention. I consider positive psychology part of wellness. You have heard about positivity and negativity throughout the book. The brain's affinity to negativity as described early in the book as negativity bias and the suggestions to promote positivity at times seem at odds and I want to revisit a few important points, while adding new ones.

Generally I will support positive psychology with a few caveats. Many authors write inspirationally about positive psychology. It is an important focus of my work with cancer patients to assist them in discovering strategies to focus on emotions and thoughts that they experience as healthy and desirable. I will, however, always remind you that we are individuals and that some approaches work better for some and other approaches for others. There are data showing that people with a negative self-image get worse if you force them into positive thinking. What is right for the goose is not always right for the gander. But as long as shifting emotion and thought towards positivity does not make you feel worse, let me state my case for positivity.

When I say positivity, I include the absence of negativity. You have already seen this. I will encourage you not only to increase the positive but to decrease something negative. Positive, aka happiness and relaxation, is good for you. The same way ongoing distress (notice that I did not say stress) can do bad stuff to you, happiness can do good stuff to you.

But remember that decreasing the negative stuff does not mean to suppress negative emotions. On the contrary. I quoted Susan David earlier that showing up for your emotion is an important prerequisite that allows you to more easily "step out" of emotions and not be consumed by them. She further argues that "unless we can process, navigate, and be comfortable with the full range of our emotions, we won't learn to be resilient" and to "tell ourselves to 'think positive' and to push negative or difficult emotions aside won't work" (Semnani, *Washington Post*, September 23, 2016). This distinction is important!

We discussed how cancer patients are often worried about being stressed and not being happy. Many are distressed about being distressed. By now many people know that stress and depressive mood can have a negative impact not just on their well-being but on their physical health. There are numerous studies to show that. I assume most everybody is on board to decrease negativity and increase positivity as long as that process is not stressful in itself. No one is negating the importance of happiness, we're just debating how to best get there.

Happiness leads to better marriage, health, friendship, creativity, and careers. Shawn Achor in his book, *The Happiness Advantage*, gives numerous examples and advocates small steps. I very much support and encourage cancer patients to do the same. It is not just the 10,000 hours of practice that make you proficient at something. You can change emotion, body state, and thoughts in small steps and (to reiterate Dan Harris) gradually. What is even better, you can change emotion, thoughts, and body within minutes. What can feel frozen and static can become fluid. One minute we have one experience, and the next it is different. Life is not static, but like emotions and thoughts, it ebbs and flows.

I support the pursuit of happiness. You can re-read about its importance in *The Happiness Track* by Emma Seppälä, which I mentioned earlier. It makes you learn faster, think more creatively, and resolve challenging situations better. Positive emotions help you bounce back from stress more quickly. Happiness strengthens existing relationships. Shared laughter makes people more open and willing to cooperate. Happiness increases productivity and commitment in the workplace. It increases strength, coordination, sleep, and immune function. The list is endless.

What I see, however, and Seppälä's book points it out, is that people get distressed by the absence of happiness and the presence of distress. In their obsessive pursuit of happiness as Ruth Whippman describes so beautifully in her book *America the Anxious*, people become nervous wrecks. I encourage you to pursue happiness since it has many benefits, but don't get distressed by the pursuit, or if you do, address the distress around happiness before you address happiness. If you notice the absence of happiness or the presence of distress, take small steps in the right direction.

Okay, so I have made my case for promoting positivity *as long as you do not get sucked into the "happiness fad."* What ultimately convinced me are the effects of positivity itself. Ian Gotlib is the Director of the Stanford Neurodevelopment, Affect, and Psychopathology (SNAP) Laboratory. I had heard about his research many years ago, and it blew me away. I am interested in child development, and he presented a study that I found remarkable. He recruited non-depressed daughters from mothers who themselves were depressed. He set up a computer task for the girls and let them look at images with sad and happy faces. He compared these non-depressed girls whose mothers were depressed with non-depressed girls whose mothers were not depressed. Keep in mind that none of these girls themselves were depressed!

What Gotlib and his collaborators found was that the non-depressed girls from depressed mothers were more likely to focus on sad faces compared to the non-depressed girls from non-depressed mothers (Joormann et al., 2007). It is another perfect illustration of "incognito." Even though the girls were not depressed themselves, they tended to have attentional bias towards sad facial expressions and didn't even realize it. Fortunately the study also showed that non-depressed girls from depressed mothers could be taught to change that negative attentional bias naturally by looking at positive stimuli rather than negative ones (LeMoult et al., 2016).

Since 40 percent of children of affectively ill parents will become depressed by the age of twenty (Beardslee et al., 1998), effective preventive measures are imperative, and I will hopefully find a study one day that shows that bias interventions will help adolescents to not advance to depression as their parents did.

Oh, and please don't think Professor Gotlib discriminates against adolescent boys. He simply picked girls because unfortunately there are more women with depression and it was easier to recruit.

But we don't have to wait for the results of preventive studies to know that positive stimulation is good for us. It is true that prevention is best. It is also true that early intervention is good. And I also follow the motto "Better late than never" and "Never say never." I strongly believe that change is possible at any time. Work from Gotlib's lab in collaboration with researchers from

Canada and Michigan confirms that. You heard about this study already when I talked about attention restoration (a fancy word to say to give the brain a break). If you look at depressed people who take a stroll in nature versus an urban setting, the ones who take a walk in nature will improve their mood, and even better, their memory improves, too (Berman et al., 2012).

The importance of what your eyes see is fundamental for cancer patients. I asked you already not to slouch, but I will now also ask you to rest your eyes on pleasant images and breathe out slowly whenever you can. I will now add: let your eyes rest on something nature related. And it does not mean you have to get out of bed.

Everybody will encourage you to take a walk while you are dragging during treatment because "it is good for you." Nope. Not necessarily. If you have the energy, sure, a walk is good, but when you cannot get out of bed because of fatigue or nausea, then a walk is not appropriate. But get a little bonsai or let your eyes rest on a screensaver tree or watch the Nature channel during chemotherapy.

Remember that surgical patients left the hospital faster when their room faced the courtyard compared to a busy street in front of the hospital (Ulrich, 1984). Looking at nature works without you even moving a toe. Cognitive scientists might argue this last point as they claim that the environment in which you restore needs to be reasonably large (like a walk in the woods) and needs to give you the feeling of being away (Kaplan & Berman, 2010). A cancer patient, however, does not always have that luxury. We've got to work with what is realistic and feasible.

EGO CONGRUENCY

I have presented you with scientific evidence that supports many of my clinical observations and the exercises and meditations I suggest as a result. There is, however, an observation that I make repetitiously with clients that I haven't found an explanation for in the scientific literature. When patients have an insight that feels true to them, I often observe a visible sense of relief. There is what from the outside looks like a settling or relaxation of body and mind. It is physically discernible. I call it ego-congruency or ego-synchronicity.

Patients have described it as a physical internal "drop." It is a form of being in sync or in tune with oneself.

This congruency is what I described earlier about the people with a negative self-image who get worse if you force them into positive thinking. If you confront your thought about yourself "I am not good enough" with someone else's reassurance that "you are good enough," it creates an incongruence with oneself that results in the described negative change in affect. It is my experience that it is easier to change when we at first fully embrace our inner reality, even if our particular reality is something that most people would view as only negative.

I remember a patient who had fought all her life against her family background. She had come from challenging circumstances. Her mother was a sex worker, her father an alcoholic. Even though she grew up in a loving adoptive family, she could never quite shake the sense that she was "no good." She had worked very hard all her life to compensate for feeling not good enough. It was not until the day she broke down and started repetitiously saying, "I am no good, I am no good" that she felt a sense of relief. Owning her personal truth led to a cathartic relief. Anybody who has watched Emma Thompson's 2022 movie *Good luck to You, Leo Grande* can appreciate the societal contributions of sex workers, but this didn't help this patient to shake her belief about the reputation of that profession and how it had affected her sense of self.

There seems to be a disconnect between what we rationally "know" and what we incognitoly (I just have declared incognito a verb and adjective) "know." Once she could admit to herself that she was "no good," she was finally able to change from within by truly changing a belief that she had rationally known for a long time to be incorrect but could only defend against and could only compensate for by being successful.

Figure 4

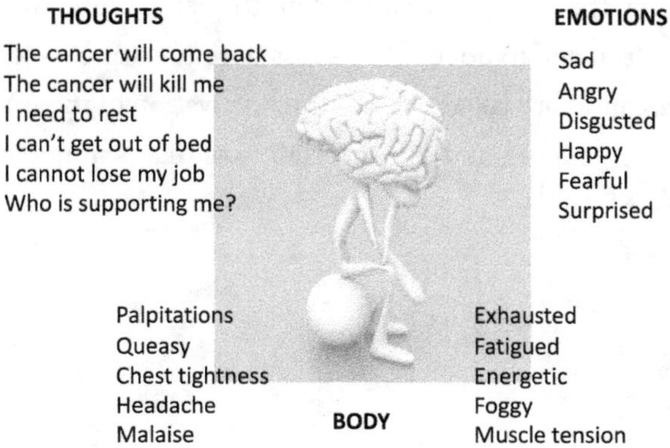

There is another cancer-relevant aspect of the idea that body and mind are ONE that I want to discuss. Remember Figure 4? Here it is again. Cancer patients have a lot of physical symptoms. Sometimes it is very hard to separate cancer or cancer treatment-related physical symptoms from stress activation-based physical symptoms. ANS activation causes physical symptoms that can also be caused by cancer.

How is a patient supposed to differentiate between a tension headache that is stress based and one that is caused by a cancer metastasis? How are you supposed to not get scared by nausea if that was the presenting symptom of your stomach cancer, even if everybody is telling you that it is "just stress."

Jordan had a rare cancer located in his upper abdomen. It happened to be situated close to where he would consistently experience pressure and pain. He naturally decided that the discomfort was related to the tumor. It also happened to be situated close to his solar plexus, which is part of the autonomic nervous system.

After a while Jordan noticed that stress would exacerbate the symptoms. He learned to decrease the discomfort through breathing exercises and relaxation. At that point, he realized that the discomfort was not related to the tumor, but the pain was evoked by activation of the sympathetic tone. It could easily have been the other way around, however. Tumors do press on nerves and other body structures and can cause considerable pain. It is not always easy to know the difference. It is always very important to keep in mind that the cancer itself maybe the culprit and to not easily dismiss symptoms as caused by distress. But after all other causes are ruled out, consider activation of the ANS as a possible cause. Both are possible, and the uncertainty of that is unnerving.

CHAPTER 8.

The Concept of Human Needs

In the preceding chapters, I have been establishing a theoretical framework and laying a foundation for you to accept that there is complexity and difficulty in how to change your thinking and your emotional experiences as well as your body state. But that it is possible! Change does not come as easily as most of us would like, but these *are* learnable skills. And an important ingredient and prerequisite are our most inner motivations and core values.

We have looked at sudden versus gradual change and the different levels of control or lack of control that we have over our cells. Lasting change takes practice, and I have already introduced you to several exercises to help this process. I have also embedded exercises along the way to assure practice with expanding awareness.

Insight is presumably the first step to change, but as many of us know, we can have many insights over time, and they do not necessarily result in behavior change. We often have insights and don't act on them. We know we should live with moderation, for example, or exercise and eat healthy but still find ourselves doing late night snacking or thinking about that we *should* walk rather than actually going out and doing it. By now you know to use the word "should" when you hear it externally or in your head only as an inspiration to go deeper and explore what motivates you and understand the factors that can truly help and support you.

So if insight is not enough, what else do we need? I am convinced that it is fundamental to understand the often not or only partially conscious needs and motivations that drive our behavior. These are often contrary to the more rational insights we have. If cookies give you comfort, the knowledge that you should only eat them in moderation will not be enough to actually eat them in moderation.

In the process of uncovering these needs and motivations, I will often tell patients that understanding the reason for non-action is as valuable as understanding the motivation for action. We might have insight into why we want to do things, but many of us have little insight into why we *don't* do certain things that seem rationally so obvious. Unearthing those mysterious driving forces can be very helpful in facilitating change.

NEEDS AND WANTS

Needs and *wants* are words I used on the first few pages of the book, but I want to make sure we share the same understanding of what they signify. As I mentioned on those first pages, "need" means different things to different people in different contexts. I have turned to word definitions on Google regularly, not always to take them at face value, as they often lack depth and accuracy but as a starting point to stimulate thought. I am intrigued by their definition for "need": *a thing that is wanted or required.* This definition reveals just how easy it is to get into trouble as we apply different meanings to the same word. *Wanted* and *required* are hardly interchangeable! Such a definition also highlights that some needs can be fundamental for survival while others are mental constructs that we build around "soft" needs.

Bear with me here.

When I am with a patient, am I talking to someone who "wants" their doctor to listen to them, or am I talking to someone who "requires" that their doctor listen to them? The very idea of a "need" moves on a continuum with respect to the necessity to fulfill it, and we have to define what it means to us and to the person we are communicating with. As always there is much variation. In **Chapter 1**, I touched on the fact that human experience, including health and illness, spans a wide continuum, and that we have to keep in mind that we are unique. And in the next chapter, we will look in detail at how to deal with this continuum.

The word "need" also represents a continuum—from wanting something like a new sweater to the absolutely requiring something like food or shelter and every option in between depending on circumstances and on you in those circumstances. Often a need refers simply to an important personal core value. For some it might be integrity, for others enjoyment or reliability. Take a moment to reflect on your top three core values.

I also want to alert you to the way researchers use the term "need" in the context of cancer. Providers of cancer care have long recognized that cancer patients do not have all their needs met. Researchers in Canada developed a questionnaire in the hope of capturing as many unmet needs as possible from cancer patients that had been one to five years out from their cancer (Campbell et al., 2011). Among the top ten needs they identified were dealing with fears about the cancer spreading, being told about having cancer, not feeling sure the cancer had gone, feeling tired, feeling stressed, dealing with worrying, finding information about complementary and alternative treatment, having a bad memory or lack of focus, and worry whether treatment had worked. The list is a combination of very practical things, like energy, memory, and access to some types of care, but an important common denominator is some form of worry. I applaud the authors for having taken on the arduous task of developing and validating a questionnaire to detect who needs help and what kind of help patients might need.

Since a prominent factor on the list is "worry," and worry is so very pervasive, especially with cancer, I suggest you give the following exercise a try.

Instead of saying "I am worried about cancer still being there," experiment with saying, "When I think about the cancer still being there, I feel stressed or worried because my need for ___________ is not met." What is the first word that comes to mind? The first word. Don't think too much about it. Filling in the blank, people will commonly say, "safety, control, or certainty."

Be curious about your word. This will get you out of using "worry" as an emotion, as I had advocated earlier. Instead of having a diffuse worry—"is my cancer still there"—you will have a concrete thing you can tackle—addressing your need for control/safety/certainty.

Please try to adhere to the one-word single noun practice and don't replace the word with a lengthy sentence, which is what we brainy creatures tend to do. The purpose here is to tap into motivations and needs that are not conscious or that you feel reluctant to acknowledge as true.

I have already raved about the book *Incognito* by David Eagleman. His book has convinced me that I want to capitalize on the valuable information inside of me. I hope you do also and are ready to practice diligently.

EXERCISES: CORE NEEDS

Let's build on the exercise you just did and on practices introduced in earlier chapters. We are personalizing and expanding on Mr. Baldwin's life ping-pong. The principle is the same. You take an event and see how it affects your body, your emotions, and your thought process. As I discussed in **Chapter 2** on **Advocating for Purity**, thoughts, emotions, and body are signals that serve as connectors to often unconscious information and help you recognize your needs, and they serve as the alert system that something is amiss. The event is just the trigger that gets the system "human" going.

There are numerous variations on the theme, but it goes something like this. "When I was diagnosed with cancer, I felt angry (for more emotionally oriented people) or distressed (for more physically oriented people) because my need for (blank) was not met." Figure 9 gives you a visual of the procedure.

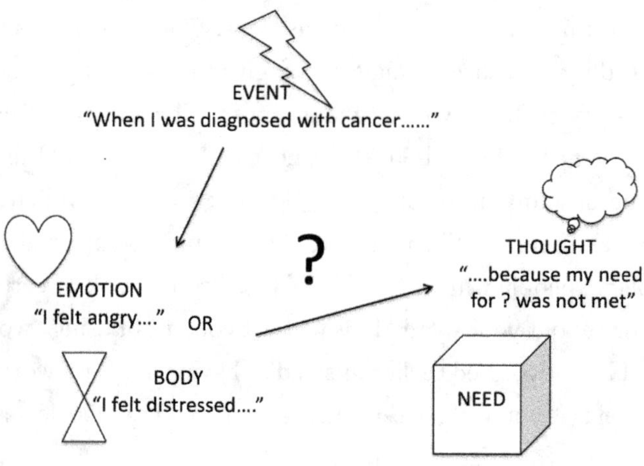

Figure 9

Valuable information stems from filling in this blank. Common words people will use are safety, control, closeness, certainty, etc. *When I was diagnosed with cancer, I felt angry because my need for safety was not met.* Instead of fixating on the monster "diagnosis of cancer," we can focus on how to satisfy the need—for safety, control, closeness, certainty, etc. Strangely enough the body tends to settle and calm when important needs are met.

When life does not allow you to meet a particular need, your body can be placated by meeting another need. You can even consider not having to fulfill the originally perceived need. In the section **Needs Exercise Algorithm** ahead, you will find several scenarios that walk you through this principle to give you practice. Susan David, the Harvard psychologist I mentioned in **Chapter 5** on **Emotions**, makes a similar suggestion. She wants you to cultivate habits that are congruent with your values of what she calls "want-to goals." A want-to goal is a change that is driven by your values as opposed to a "have-to goal" that is externally imposed. When we pursue actions that are based in our values and needs, our emotions follow and generally lift and feel lighter, and our thoughts become more flexible and creative.

In **Chapter 4** on **Thinking,** I already discussed the rigidity with which our thoughts tend to hang around, but that rigidity is not limited just to thinking. Think about the rigidity with which we at times insist on meeting our needs. It can feel as if it is the only thing that will do. I am sure you have experienced the intensity of wanting something very badly with your—or even particularly with your—loved ones. But it does not have to be that way.

By the way, when I talk here about the need for *control*, please don't think I am accusing anyone of being a "control freak." I'm simply talking about having a sense of mastery, charge, and agency of whatever is happening to you at any given time.

You can try this core needs-identifying exercise with other aspects of your life. "When <u>my partner did not cook dinner</u> [the event], I felt <u>disappointed</u> [emotion] because my need for <u>support</u> was not met [core need]." Here we are not assigning blame to the partner or questioning his/her motives in not cooking dinner, we're simply discovering that support is something that sustains us and would have been nice to get. As life would have it, sometimes we can receive it, sometimes we have to live without it. Through this exercise, you identify what's beneath your disappointment (and perhaps won't be so quick to yell at your partner for not cooking, though in your weaker moments you will do that also, and I'll help you forgive yourself for it).

Before we figure out how you can get dinner or other support or alternatively crawl into bed to watch TV instead, let us pause. Let's consider your options and consider them carefully. In **Chapter 5** on **Emotions,** I had introduced you to the book *Nonviolent Communication* by Marshall Rosenberg. In his book, Rosenberg offers an "emotions" list, and he also provides a "needs" list. I have compiled a list of needs that I have collected from my work with patients. Readers of Rosenberg's work will notice that my list shares components with his, but I curated my list, so it contains the words most relevant and common to cancer patients. It is by no means exhaustive. I have left some room at the end, so you can add your own words. And it is printed on a separate page, so you can easily make a copy to carry around with you or copy to your phone, so it will be easily accessible when you get stuck in daily life.

List of needs

Acceptance	Accommodation	Accuracy	Affection
Appearance	Appreciation	Attention	Authenticity
Autonomy	Awareness	Belonging	Calmness
Caring	Caregiving	Certainty	Challenge
Choice	Clarity	Closeness	Collaboration
Comfort	Commitment	Communication	Community
Companionship	Compassion	Competence	Completion
Comprehension	Conduct	Confidence	Connection
Consideration	Consistency	Contentment	Contribution
Control	Courage	Courtesy	Creativity
Depth	Ease	Effectiveness	Efficiency
Empathy	Enjoyment	Engagement	Entertainment
Enthusiasm	Equality	Excitement	Experience
Fairness	Freedom	Fun	Growth
Harmony	Health	Honesty	Hope
Humor	Identity	Independence	Innovation
Insight	Integrity	Intelligence	Intimacy
Joy	Justice	Kindness	Knowledge
Learning	Longevity	Love	Manageability
Mastery	Maturity	Meaning	Moderation
Modesty	Mutuality	Novelty	Nurturing
Nurturing	Opportunity	Order	Playfulness
Pleasure	Practicality	Presence	Precision
Preparedness	Prioritization	Privacy	Propriety
Punctuality	Purpose	Reality	Relationship
Relevance	Reliability	Respect	Safety
Security	Sincerity	Space	Spontaneity
Stability	Stimulation	Success	Support
Synergy	Thoughtfulness	Tolerance	Trust
Truthfulness	Understanding	Validity	Value
Warmth	Worthiness		

Figure 10

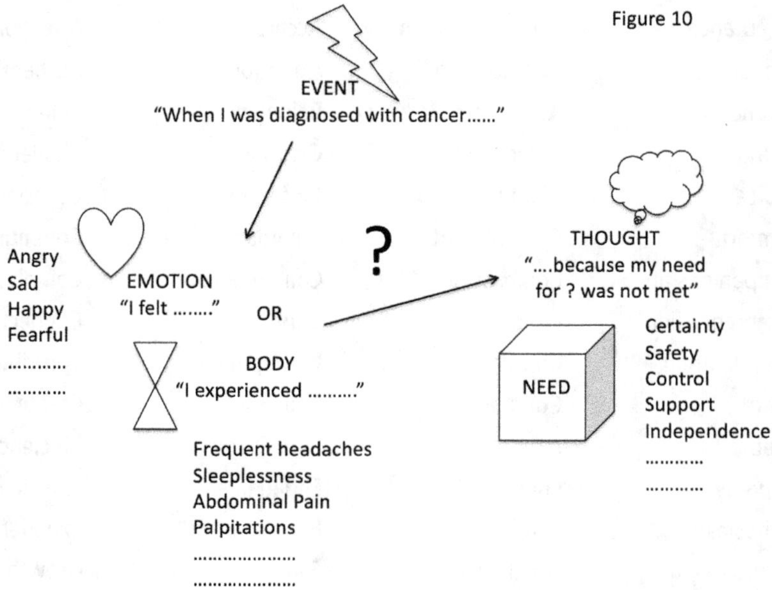

Looking at Figure 10, you will recognize "event, emotion, and thought" from **Chapter 3**, where we discussed how our body processes events. We discussed William James's (and other peoples') notion of what happens to your thinking and emotions when a lion (or in your situation the cancer) is the event. The "need" box, however, is familiar from Rosenberg's concept. Figure 10 is the practice version of Figure 9. It blends the different ideas into one practice.

Try it for yourself. I offer some options, but there are empty lines for you to fill in your own experience. And of course, you get to use whatever event you want as I described at the beginning of this core need exercise section.

EVENTS, EMOTIONS, THOUGHTS, AND NEEDS

The following exercise was also inspired by Rosenberg's book. Rosenberg teaches us to take responsibility for our emotions and be precise in expressing them. As we practice doing this, our ability to be precise grows and deepens awareness and enhances our interactions with others.

You'll recall that Rosenberg discourages using words like "abandoned, ignored, pressured, threatened, rejected, or betrayed" to describe our emotions.

These words imply that the emotion has an external origin or cause; the word "threatened" implies that someone did something to make you feel a certain way. Notice how the sentence "I feel threatened by my cancer" has a very different ring to it than "I feel scared because my need for safety and certainty is not met." We'll be practicing using this kind of precision to describe the emotions we're experiencing. At first you might feel a little foolish or think your language sounds stilted. But I can assure you that putting a non-judgmental twist to Mr. Baldwin's ping-pong with life can be very liberating.

We acquire and we habituate to our personal language usually from the people who raise us. Social psychologists inform us that language development works better if we feel positively attached to the person from whom we learn it (Assous et al., 2018), but even if we don't have the privilege of positive attachment, the language we use feels as if it is ours. When we start to change the words we use to express ourselves, the new phrases do not run in the grooves we've spent a lifetime establishing. But after a while of practice, the different words can feel freeing. Not unlike the feel of learning any new language, where we gradually and with lots of practice transition from stringing words into stilted sentences to letting words easily roll off our tongue.

I laughingly remember how I went mute for three weeks after taking a workshop with Marshall Rosenberg. All of my "emotion" words were on the page of no-nos. I literally walked around with a piece of paper in my pocket that I had copied from his book to help me figure out exactly what I was feeling. So don't get discouraged if you discover that you are not an emotion master. You can learn, and if you don't enjoy the process, if you are what I would call "non-feeler," I will offer an alternative solution.

You might have noticed that the second sentence above, "I feel scared because my need for safety and certainty is not met," does not contain the word cancer. If you remove the word "cancer," it helps you realize that it is not just the cancer itself that causes trouble in your body but that the experience with cancer evokes a lack of safety and certainty—or whatever need might be threatened for you. This is the reason I had you internalize Mr. Baldwin's response to the car cutting in front of him as your constant mental companion.

Yes, cancer sucks, but if you realize that important needs are not met as part of the experience with cancer, you have more leverage to create a sense of well-being despite having cancer. It is often less scary to go after needs than to go after cancer. You feel a better sense of control, and as you have heard me say several times now, humans like that. Cancer is still the competitor to deal with, but as you become better able to identify precisely what you need, you will feel more in charge of addressing your cancer and needs.

COULD THOUGHTS REPRESENT NEEDS?

Take another look at Figure 10. Do you see how closely I position the "thought cloud" with the "need box?" I have already argued in **Chapter 4** on **Thinking** that many thoughts can be interpreted as stand-ins for needs. I want to reiterate the notion that "needs" can be viewed as a form of thought. I suspect some of you will resist this idea, and I don't know if any researchers share my opinion, but I have found the idea useful with my patients.

It is true that we have basic needs, such as food and shelter for our survival, but when we get into the more abstract concepts of human needs, I can make a case that needs are intellectual concepts. Do we really "need" support, understanding, autonomy, and love the same way we need food and shelter?

I want to draw an analogy to our earlier discussion of basic emotions and secondary emotions (**Chapter 5**). We cannot prevent feeling angry or sad. The body will just produce that emotion because of our evolutionary development, as I noted there. Similarly we have little control over our need for calories and sleep. The body will demand them. But we can probably muster a little more flexibility with the need for understanding and support. It is in fact our rigidity in insisting on fulfilling needs that often gets us in trouble.

Indeed fulfilling needs is central to human existence and helps us sustain life. Here I want to suggest that you could consider tolerating not always being able to satisfy all needs. Finding a balance between pursuing the fulfillment of needs and tolerating their absence can contribute to balance and well-being. It is my clinical observation that patients in distress have a tendency to pursue their core needs more vigorously (than those of us not similarly distressed), often without success, and thus adding considerable distress to their system.

As distress comes with a decrease in cognitive ability and flexibility as we learned earlier (in **Chapter 4** on **Thinking** and **Chapter 6** on **Body**), you have to make provisions to maintain some flexibility to be at your best when you take on cancer.

While it is human to resort to what is most familiar when we are distressed, we also need to be realistic about whether or not it is feasible to fulfill those needs. Since the body is pretty agreeable and not as demanding as the mind, we can often pacify it with other means. There are also techniques to pacify the body without satisfying needs, as I described earlier (in the section about the autonomic nervous system in **Chapter 6** on **Body**). A few breaths in the absence of negative thought never hurt.

I will offer suggestions for how to work with this observation about rigidity around needs and possible alternatives in the following section on developing your personal algorithms.

FLEXIBILITY AND RIGIDITY OF NEEDS

I want to discuss in more depth what I just called rigidity around fulfilling your needs when you are distressed. I am sure social psychologists have studied extensively why we continue behavior that does not serve us or the situation we are in. My clinical observation in a cancer context is that people tend to use the coping strategies that they are best at or were most comfortable with before they got ill. I think there are different reasons for this.

One reason is that humans like familiarity, even when it comes at a price. We tend not to want to step out of our comfort zone. As we know from abusive relationships with people and substances, we stay with what is familiar, even if it is not good for us. Here I remind you of my friend's quote from early on that "to sit in your shit is by no means pleasant, but it is at least warm and familiar." But this inertia has clear downsides.

If you are someone who uses coping strategies of planning, control, and organization, which may work brilliantly for you in a work setting, there is a good chance that those particular strategies are not most useful for the job "cancer." But instead of making adjustments, we tend to intensify our coping strategies, even if they don't work or don't apply. If you were a planner before you got ill, you might get even more organized and show up at your doctor's appointment with a fat binder full of detailed information. Yes, sometimes it can be helpful if you are as informed as your treating team, but if searching the internet for information in an area about which you are not an expert has you feeling overwhelmed, the task can add more distress than help.

Another reason has to do with our conditioned mindsets. If you grew up in a situation where you had to be supportive of and adaptable to others, you might struggle with accepting help when you're diagnosed with cancer. It's obvious that you need help when you are sick, but if your mindset is *I need to help others*, you will have a hard time transitioning to welcome help. If your mindset is *I need to be tough*, you might judge yourself when your body demands a nap after chemotherapy.

At first glance, these situation seem to be no-brainers, but many of you know from experience what it looks like when ideas turn into fundamental needs, even if fulfilling them doesn't serve us.

Our rigidity around needs gets more pronounced when sympathetically aroused (just checking if you remember). It is important to recognize this augmentation and make adjustments. Even if you continue the behavior because you are habituated to it and get some satisfaction from it, also consider delegating the research part about your cancer to someone with expertise and save your organizational skills for your closet. The body fortunately does not know the difference as long as it gets some control and organization (remember the close correlation of body and needs?). The body strangely enough settles and calms when important personal needs are met.

Figures 9 and 10 showed the stepwise instruction for how to go through the practice. I encourage you to do it step by step in the beginning, particularly if you struggle with the differentiation and identification of thought, emotion, body sensation, and identification of needs. The practice, even if it feels awkward at first, will help you develop self-awareness that will come in handy during your journey with cancer. As you start feeling comfortable with the concept or if you just want efficiency, I also offer a shortcut in Figure 11:

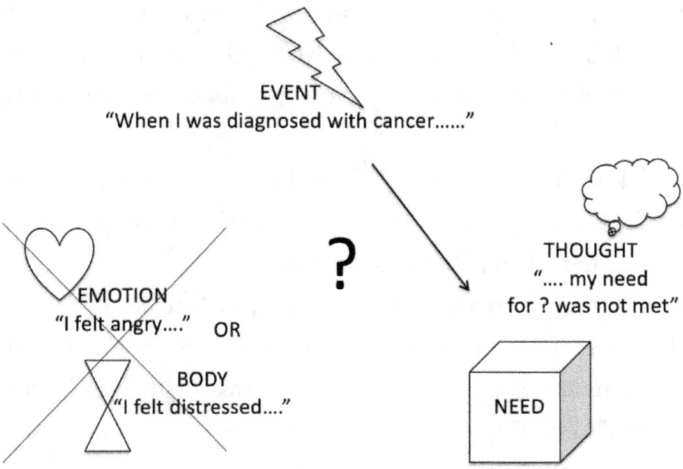

Figure 11

You get to skip the whole identification process of body and emotion! The sentence to complete here: "When I was diagnosed with cancer, my need for (blank) was not met."

At first you might hesitate about going into such a reflective, pensive state. You might feel slightly thrown off. A little puzzlement, a little hesitancy. That's because this exercise bypasses cognition. It taps straight into what I have affectionately started to call "let's go Eagleman" or "let's tap into Incognito" with my patients. It is a shortcut for this particular reflection. Turning inward. This vast internal space holds precious information about you. Accessing the answer to the question "What do I need right now" is not a process without some thought. But tapping into the relevant knowledge works better from this more dreamy, floaty state—which I have difficulty describing but which you will immediately relate to when you first experience it. It might correspond to your experience of Sharon Salzberg's description of change in **Chapter 1** or Cal Newport's uni-tasking, which I mentioned in **Chapter 4** on **Thinking**.

It is important that you let the word float to awareness on its own. I often see patients pause, with a reflective look on their face, and the word that floats to the surface takes them by surprise. That word will be more informative than if you judge the word away by exclaiming that the discovery could not possibly be true.

Try to stick with the list of single-word needs if you want the optimal benefit from the exercise. You will access the "knowing without knowing" that I talked about earlier when discussing "incognito."

But beware. If your answer to the question is, "I need the cancer to go away" or "I need a more supportive partner," you are not on the right track. It is true that you need those things, but those answers do not help you tap into "incognito." The single-word noun that comes to mind first is your best bet.

This last practice described in Figure 11 is, by the way, fulfilling my promise to provide an alternative for "non-feelers." If you struggle with identifying emotions or are simply not in the mood, you can go directly to "I need."

NEEDS EXERCISE ALGORITHM

I hope I don't sound like I want to turn everyone into self-absorbed narcissists, who only think about themselves and their needs. The main purpose of the exercise is to get insight about yourself to increase your effectiveness. This is an exercise I recommend to patients and caretakers alike. And if I were queen of the world, I would add it to the water supply of humanity. It works for EVERYBODY. With that knowledge, you can make choices based on the algorithm presented in Figure 12:

Figure 12

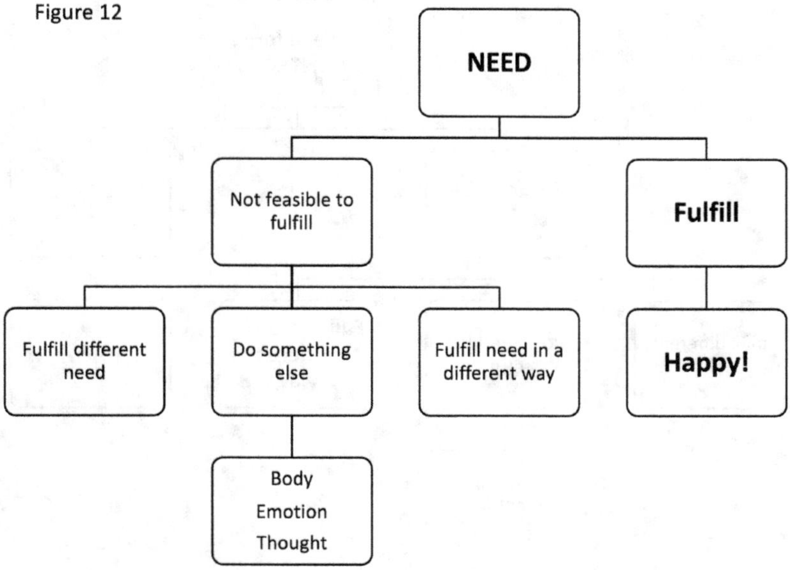

Identify a need. In a next step, you will decide whether or not it is feasible to fulfill it. If the answer is yes, you will feel happy or satisfied. Something in the overall positive category.

The next few figures walk you through your different options in more detail if it is not feasible to fulfill the particular need you want to satisfy. If it is not feasible to fulfill a need, you can satisfy a different need or fulfill the need in a different area in which it is feasible. Or you can do something altogether different. I will walk you through the different paths by marking them in bold.

I want to illustrate with some examples.

Take a look at Figure 13. You are welcome to do the exercise for any need, but for now I want to walk you through it with a defined option, just to illustrate.

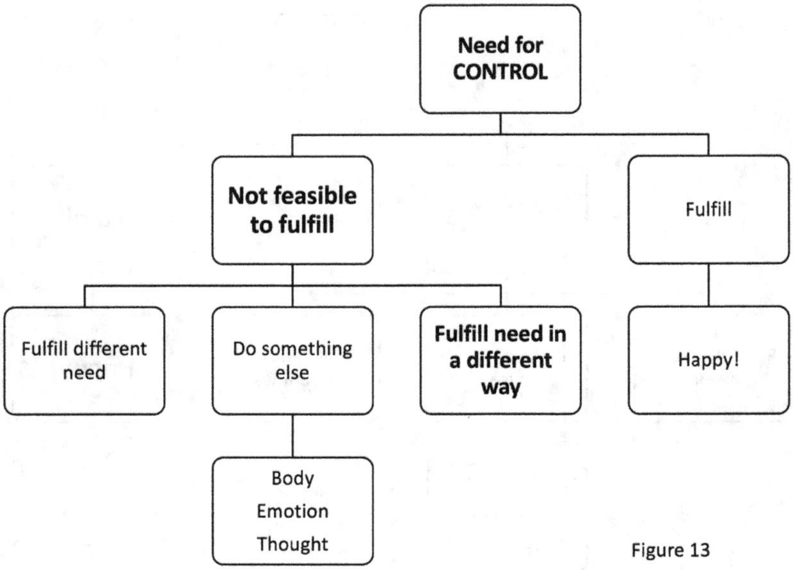

Figure 13

Try to remember a situation in which you were furious. Something set you off; it does not even matter what it was. Just assume you have identified that your need "control" was not met. If you actually do the exercise and identify a need other than "control," just replace the word in Figure 13 with your own word (common frontrunners in this case are fairness, respect, and feeling heard or understood).

The next step is to assess if it is feasible to get control (or whatever need you identified) in the situation that triggered the anger (Hint: it often is not feasible to satisfy the need). Now decide if you want to satisfy the need in a different area in which it is feasible. In other words, is there an alternative activity that would give you a feeling of control? If you cannot control your doctor showing up on time, for example, can you control the process of parking, so you can arrive at the appointment not feeling stressed?

Figure 14 takes you down a different track on the algorithm. If you opt against fulfilling the need "control," either because it is not feasible or you cannot think of another activity that would represent the need for "control," then you can decide if you want to fulfill a different need. If you cannot get "control," would you settle for the alternative "organization?" At that point, you start weeding the garden or cleaning your closet. You can pick anything your heart desires.

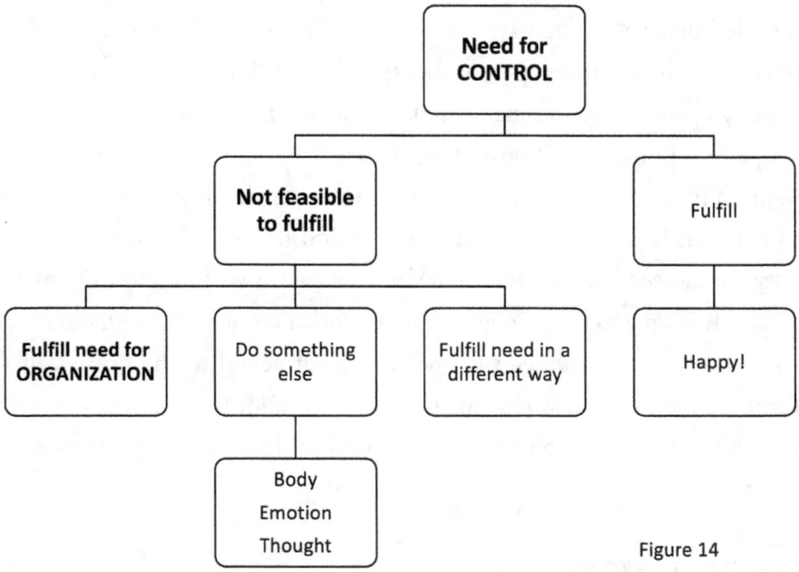

Figure 14

If you don't enjoy the whole business of dealing with needs, then as highlighted in bold in Figure 15, you can always do something else. You can always consider changing your thoughts, emotion, or body.

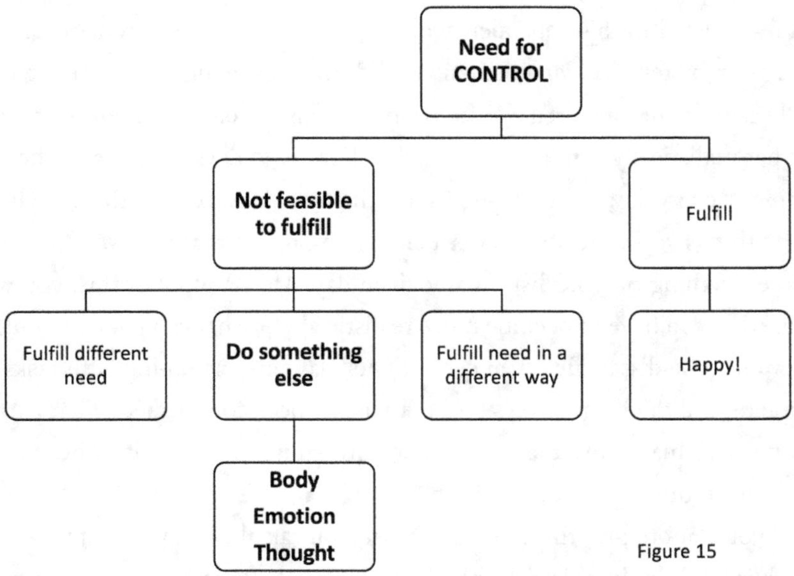

Figure 15

By now you have been introduced to many exercises to get those three into a more desirable state. You have the choice of thought replacement, generation of an emotion other than anger, or focusing on your body with any of the body exercises you have learned so far. Anything that contributes to well-being!

A patient of mine calls himself a "tinkerer." Tinkering is a perfect way to do something else that will have a high chance at yielding something that is good for you. Remember attention restoration theory? Tinkering is a good activity for cancer patients whose default brain network has a propensity to ruminate. It is a perfect way to give that network a rest and through the miracle of association, the "you" who happens to be attached to the brain will feel better. If worse comes to worst, you can always count backwards from 100 or do multiples of nine. Whatever keeps stressful, low-yield, problem-solving thought content low.

THE FEASIBILITY EXERCISE

A word on feasibility. I notice that patients get excited about the practice and are happy to try. Part of the instruction about feasibility, however, often gets lost in translation. I am not sure why we humans have a tendency to bang our head against the wall, even if it is made of concrete and not penetrable. I suspect it is related to this dependency on clinging to needs that are familiar and core to our existence. Giving them up would constitute a threat to our existence.

Feasibility has inspired the following exercise: Take a moment to reflect on what realistically can be done in a day. For seven days running, at the beginning of every day, write a to-do list for that day. At the end of the day, check off the things you were able to do. I am willing to bet that you were not able to do everything on your list on any given day. After a week of this, you will realize that you have to become more realistic about what can get done unless you want to be dissatisfied. Cancer patients' days are brimming with tasks to complete, and the list is always longer than can be accomplished. That part is real, but let's make sure that you are not drowning in tasks but rather tackle them within the bounds of feasibility.

If you want to give this exercise a twist, you can also ask yourself what can *peacefully* be done in a day? Particularly when we overestimate what can be done in a day, we have a tendency to rush through the day to get everything done, which can add a lot of distress.

THE CAN, WANT, MUST, AND SHOULD EXERCISE

Take a moment and reflect on what you are capable of doing. Physically and emotionally. These are the "CANS."

"I can walk to the mailbox. I can do the dishes. I can make my bed." Remember, "I can" literally refers to what you are capable of doing.

Now try "I want to…": "I want to play the piano. I want to climb Mount Everest. I want to win the Nobel prize. I want to write a postcard to my friend." "WANT" refers to all the things you desire and can cover the whole gamut from possible to impossible to fulfill. You might want to climb Mount Everest, but while you are being treated for cancer, that will not happen, regardless of your wanting it (because your body can't). "MUST" refers to activities that really are necessary, that will get you in trouble within a certain time period unless you execute them. Not paying your rent won't get you in trouble the next day but will cause problems within a few weeks. And then there are the "SHOULDS"—a category of thoughts that I have been trying to get out of your head since the first pages of this book. As you know, however, many of our heads are full of these "should" thoughts, and we have to deal with them. Make four columns and list all the things in the four categories that come to mind spontaneously.

Table 3 contains a few examples to illustrate my point, but I want you to create your own chart or fill in the empty boxes with your own ideas.

WANT	CAN	MUST	SHOULD
Get married	Walk to the mailbox	Pay the rent	Ride my bike
Be alive for my son's high school graduation	Take a breath		Meditate
Climb Mount Everest	Wash a plate		Not be stressed
Witness the birth of my first grandchild	Brush my teeth		Eat healthy
A hamburger			

The information in the table is often illuminating. The "want" column often is an interesting blend of bucket list items mixed with dreams and heart desires. When you think about them, you will feel various levels of emotions depending on how realistic they are to fulfill. Take that column both as an inspiration and a reality check.

Something else you will notice is that there is a huge disconnect between "can" and "should." Patients often feel they "should" exercise when they can barely make it to the fridge to get a glass of water. I strongly encourage you to do items on the "can" list.

If you are low on energy and want to feel better, simply pick something from the "can" list and get it done, however small it might be. Sometimes this exercise can jump start you into feeling more energy or improve your mood. In alignment with what you learned in **Chapter 2** on **Thought-Body-Emotion: A Love-Jealousy Triangle**, you will not feel great if you focus on the "should" list since the disconnect between what you can and presumably should do is often quite large. The next chapter will teach you how to bridge the gap.

CHAPTER 9.

Everything Moves on a Continuum and What Constitutes Normal Anyway?

I have discussed at length the close connection and interaction between emotions, thoughts, and body sensations. I also introduced you to exercises on how to incorporate the ideas with variations into daily life to increase awareness and well-being. You are becoming as proficient as Mr. Baldwin at life's ping-pong or can soon read the Odyssey in ancient Greek (figuratively speaking). I have also discussed how to integrate the idea of "needs" into the framework we are working with.

Another topic I want to discuss is the term "normal." We all want to feel "normal." What most people refer to when using that word is that they want to feel well, fit in, and live by their own and general community standards. What they forget though is that our personal, individual "normal" is not "normal" in the statistical sense of the word. The misinterpretation of other people's reality often leads to contentious debates and dissonance. There is a solution to this problem, but first I will illustrate in more detail what to keep in mind when you use the word "normal."

NORMAL DISTRIBUTION AND THE BELL CURVE

An important statistical principle and mathematical tool is called normal distribution, which refers to the probability of how data points are distributed around the mean. Figure 16a shows the graphical form of the normal distribution which is called normal curve or bell curve (Figure 16a looks remotely like a bell, doesn't it?). The curve was originally named after its mathematical originator Carl Friedrich Gauss, a German mathematician who was one of the geniuses who developed the mathematical formula for the normal distribution. How it got named "normal" can fill a whole history lesson. If your brain has turned off at this point because you are someone who hated math and statistics class in high school, don't let Figure 16a deter you from reading on. The word "normal" in this book is not used to suggest that "you are not normal" as in "there is something wrong with you." Throughout the book, the word "normal" refers to "as in the majority of people." Normal means just like most everybody else, normal as in the center of the bell curve.

Figure 16a

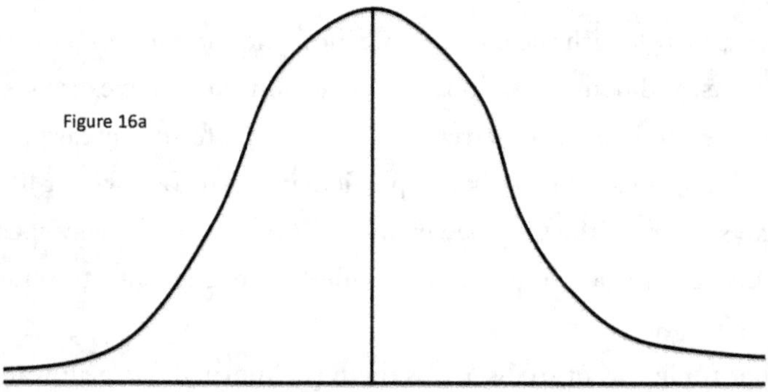

Read on about the example about height, and you will develop a better sense for the idea of the normal distribution and what it could possibly have to do with cancer. The same way I am advocating for Mr. Baldwin's lifestyle, having you dig deep into your incognito, never wanting you to forget the impact of chronic sympathetic hyperarousal, and asking that you become familiar with the idea of "needs," I am suggesting here that your life will be easier if you understand and integrate the concept of "normal distribution."

The average height of a U.S. male adult is about 5'9". This means that the majority of U.S. mens' height will lie between 5'7" and 5'11". Yes, there are many men who are 5'5" or 6'5", but they are a minority. The numbers indicate that there are less people who are very short or very tall. The statistical details and accuracy of this example are not important, but the principle is.

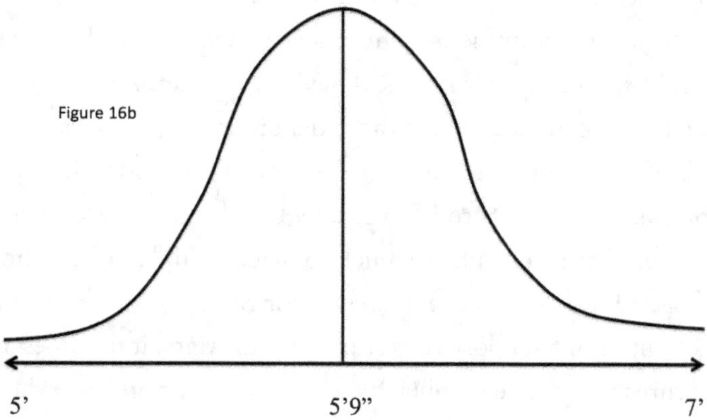

Figure 16b

When we apply this idea of normal distribution to human characteristics, it gets a little trickier because there is much more subjectivity than with height. Height is measurable, but is the trait responsibility similarly so? Most people are reasonably responsible. Then there are the famous slackers and the super responsible people on the ends of the spectrum. The slacker might not see himself as a slacker and might call the super responsible one rigid. The point is that "normal distribution" makes a statement about a feature that applies to a majority.

A considerable amount of subjectivity is involved in taking a characteristic and trying to place it on the bell curve. This can cause heated debate and considerable conflict, which the following example will illustrate. Remember the book *Men Are from Mars, Women Are from Venus*? Even though it was published in 1992, I still hear people refer to at least the idea, even if they have never read the book. The title has become a catch phrase to remind us of differences between women and men. Like height we can still fairly easily relate to the clarity of the difference of gender (and as we more and more accept that gender is not as a binary as many want it to be), but what about definitions of privacy or closeness? These are characteristics that are much more subject to individual interpretation. This is the area where it gets particularly precarious. One of the public eavesdropping clips in the *San Francisco Chronicle* drives this point home humorously. "I'm not bossy. I'm just aggressively helpful," is a woman overheard saying at a café in Berkeley. This relativity in perception is something many cancer patients have to contend with.

I often hear disappointment from cancer patients about how the people around them respond to their illness. They'll say something like, "I thought Mary would be there for me." What the patient is expressing is disappointment for the lack of expected availability or support of a friend. The situation is often as follows: Mary wants to be available, but she is so scared of seeing or hearing the word "cancer," sadly so much so that she "did not hear the phone" when Suzy asks for a ride to the hospital. For Suzy the ride to the hospital would be an important supportive gesture, but for Mary, it becomes an insurmountable threat. If you remember the concept of "incognito," Mary might not even be conscious of her fear. She might tell Suzy that she has an appointment she could not move, but to make matters worse, Suzy then sees Mary at their local coffee shop during the requested timeframe.

Suzy had always thought of Mary as responsible but is now puzzled and disappointed in her friend for what she presumes is Mary slacking off. This is just one variation of the theme.

In this situation, what either of them would have to consider about the other is that distress alters our behavior and our ability to think. When tolerance would be helpful, we have even less because we are under stress. We need to learn not to assume that how we operate is how everyone else operates.

There is a beautifully written section in Andrew Solomon's book, *The Noonday Demon*, that demonstrates how differently we can approach identical experiences. Solomon eloquently describes overhearing a woman describe how, to avoid taking medication, she has limited her life by eliminating most stimulation that could evoke depressive symptoms, whereas the author himself chooses to be on several medications to be able to tolerate and live life to the fullest extent possible.

Here are two people on the opposite end of the spectrum with respect to their desire to take medication. To develop tolerance for individual differences becomes a necessity at a time when we are least capable of being tolerant.

Often you will not recognize these differences as simply differences the same way you are capable of recognizing height and eye color without projecting judgment that brown eyes are better than blue eyes. As soon as your own needs are at stake, your personal need for control or certainty might seem reasonable and "normal" to you but seems over the top to someone else. The inability to see one's own preference for what it is, a personal preference, can become a major conflict between you and the people around you during the battle with cancer.

MORE PRACTICAL WORK ON THE CONTINUUM

The following exercises facilitate assessing yourself with respect to how you fit on the continuum compared to other people. The information from the exercise can assist you in your interactions with yourself and others.

The first exercise serves to help you evaluate your own core needs and how not having these needs fulfilled may affect your sense of self and identity. To start pick five values or characteristics that are fundamental to you as a person, such as reliability, connection, closeness, precision, privacy, and humor or whatever they might be. If nothing comes to mind spontaneously, you can let your eyes glide over the "needs" page on page 167 and let "incognito" speak to you. Some words might draw you in more than others. On some your eyes might rest before you move on. Once you have settled on five words, randomly pick one of the five.

Place yourself on the continuum of a bell curve. Remember that this exercise is designed to help you assess where you fit in comparison to other people. For example, if wanting closeness is one of the traits important to you, ask yourself how you compare to others in this desire. Do you need more closeness than your neighbors, friends, or family? If yes place a dot somewhere on the right side of the curve, representing that you are among a minority group of people who on average need more closeness than others.

This exercise requires a considerable amount of honesty with yourself. When you doubt your own judgment (or even just out of curiosity), ask two or more trusted people to assess you separately without you prompting them with your opinion about yourself. Prior to explaining the exercise to them, you can even take a moment and guess how they will assess you. Then go on to explain the principle of a normal distribution in the statistical sense and ask them to place you on the curve with the respective characteristic you are exploring: "How do you rate my need for closeness on a bell curve?"

If there is a big difference between how you assess yourself and how others assess you, it might be time for some introspection. Comparing your own view, your view of how others see you, and their own view of your need for closeness might look like Figure 17:

Figure 17

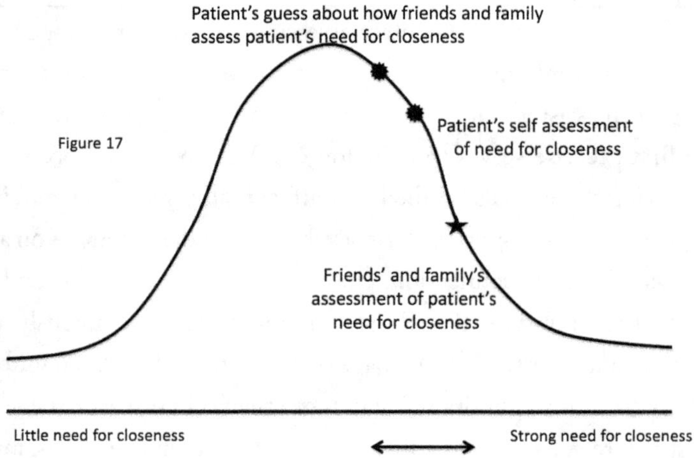

While you recognize that your need for closeness is above average compared to other people, you don't think that others view you that way, when in fact their view of you is the opposite, which is represented by the star. They think that you need more closeness than you think you do. These differences in perception lead to a distance on the bell curve, which is shown with the double arrow.

For the sake of argument, I presented an example in which the patient does not realize that others experience them as needing a lot of closeness. To make matters worse, they even misjudge the view of others about them. The take home message: the bigger the distance on the curve, the bigger the probability of trouble. If at first the exercise does not help clarify your situation, at least it will make for a lively dinner conversation about perception and interpretation!

The next exercise serves to detect whether your needs have changed during the course of your illness. You will self-assess your need for closeness or whatever you have decided to self-assess before you got ill. Then you will assess whether it has changed as the result of cancer. Your assessment might look like Figure 18:

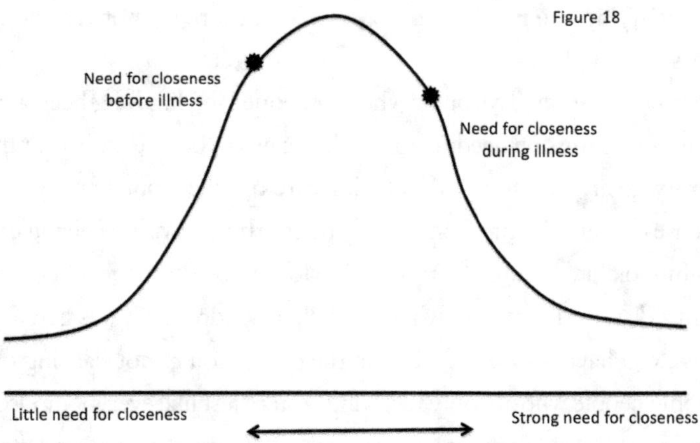

You believe that your need for closeness was slightly below average before you got sick. You enjoyed intimate conversation but would just as easily go off into the woods by yourself. But these days, you consider yourself clingy. The illness has changed your needs. You are now slightly above average compared to others. You are still within what is considered normal for the majority of people, but you have experienced a shift on the curve. If you experience such a shift, there is a very good chance that you will experience distress while going through cancer. The distress will be proportional to the number of shifted or expanded needs and the distance on the curve between how you were before cancer and how you are now.

The problem is that you might not realize that what you want is more closeness or intimacy, but you might change your behavior accordingly and take actions that reflect wanting more closeness. You might, for instance, ask someone to go shopping with you, even though you have always declared that you hate shopping. The recipient of the request might be puzzled, wondering why their beloved partner has all of a sudden become what they, too, would call clingy. Or you might notice that you have changed and hate the change. You might always have prided yourself on being independent and are upset with the person you have become. Cuddling up on the sofa with someone? No way!

Unless you become aware that your set of needs, or even only one need, has changed, you will likely face trouble or conflict. If you don't know how to go about satisfying the need or tolerate its loss, there is another good chance for distress.

One way this often plays out is when someone who has long been a caregiver suddenly becomes the one needing care. This seems to be a very difficult transition for patients who are not just used to taking care of others but actually get an important sense of their identity from it; they often struggle with receiving care. Your curve might look like Figure 19. You used to love to be there for others. It did not come from a distorted sense of giving, aka helper syndrome; it was genuine. Since your illness, you have now moved left on the curve. You're not slacking off all the way like some people who are only receiving. You're just like everybody else. Sometimes you can still do things for other people, sometimes you need others to do things for you. Normal give and take. But look at the length of the arrow. Trouble!

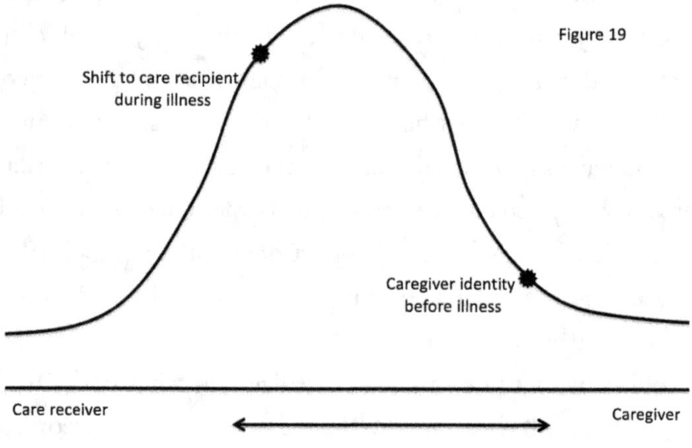

Figure 19

Let's practice our algorithm exercise to get a little more comfortable and tolerant. Remember? We have established that you cannot be a superstar caregiver. You are not willing to settle for mediocre caregiving. So caregiving is out of the picture as Figure 20 demonstrates.

What is left? Ta-daaah! Fulfill another need or do something else or fulfill the need for caregiving in a different way! Any idea? Want to glance at the needs page? Do you have a desire for excitement or mastery? Reflect what would be feasible activities to satisfy those needs. For example, climbing Mount Everest might not be the right exciting activity when you are bedbound with nausea from chemo. If you can't resist the urge to take care of something or someone and caring for your whole family is out of the question, maybe you start considering meticulous care of a house plant.

Figure 20

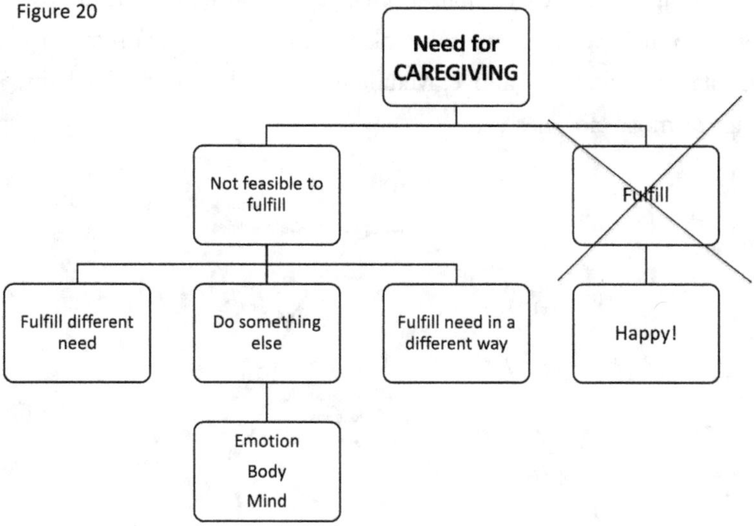

Feasibility is a fundamental aspect of the exercise. And of course, there is always good old doing something else. Write a thank you note to a friend who has helped, watch a soap on TV, or tune into the Nature channel.

This next exercise illustrates what can happen if you as the patient are not the only one who changes. We have learned that one can change during the course of illness but so can one's partner or loved ones. Or sometimes when your partners' or friends' needs always differed from yours, the distance can widen during the course of your illness, and this can add to the distress. Your curve might look like this:

The illustration in Figure 21 shows the situation of a couple, who started with different needs for closeness. While I hate to use stereotypes, the concept that *Men Are from Mars, Women Are from Venus* probably captures this best. Harold is a nice guy. He loves sports and spends his Sundays watching football. He loves to provide for his family and goes camping with his kids. His wife Maude is a teacher, very thoughtful and communicative. The couple shares a love for their children and appreciates their loyalty to each other. Before getting breast cancer, Maude didn't worry too much about the fact that she would prefer to spend more time talking with her husband and snuggling up with him watching the History Channel instead of football. But now with the cancer, even though things are going okay medically, the treatments are grueling. Looking at the curve above, Maude moves a little bit to the right. She is longing for more closeness.

Figure 21

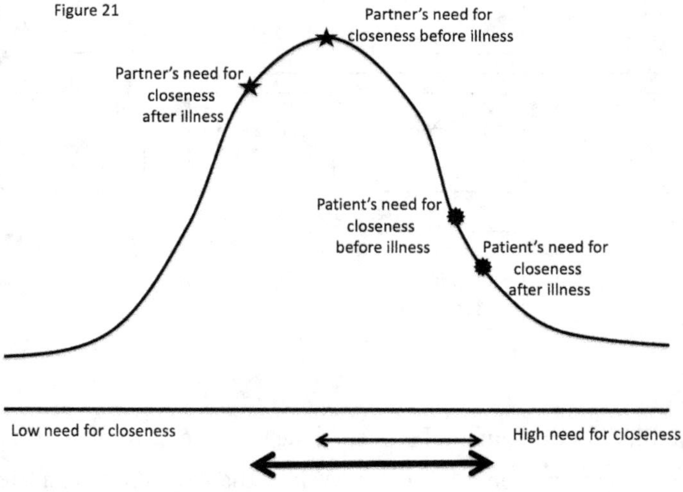

Harold is a trooper. He takes her to all her appointments. He picks up the slack with the kids, doubling his driving and cooking duty. He starts to feel worn out, and to chill, he starts watching Monday night football with a relaxing beer. Like Maude he has not changed much, but given his many duties, he has changed a bit, too. He has moved to the left on the curve. He doesn't mind a little more time to himself.

While Maude undergoes treatment, the couple gets along fine. After treatment when Maude wants to resume her previous life, she longs to spend more time with Harold, but Harold is exhausted and does not want to give up watching Monday Night Football.

Look at their curve. Even though neither of them has changed much, the bold arrow is now longer than the regular double arrow. And we have learned that if the illness results in an increased distance between the partners on the continuum of needs, they're headed for trouble.

Harold and Maude had never thought much about their differences. Now they have become apparent and a source of conflict. If you encounter such a situation in your own relationship, make sure you get help early if you can't conquer it yourself with your partner. These are situations that are fairly easy to fix if you catch them early and adapt.

COMPETING NEEDS

Chapter 8 was devoted to discussing "needs." With Harold's and Maude's story, you were unofficially introduced to the principle of competing needs, an expansion of discussing needs. In fact you have encountered it several times throughout the book. Why am I so interested in this? Let us talk about it in more detail.

Competing needs are the result of being in different places on the curve from someone else and not being able to negotiate the difference. If you look at the different examples, difficulty can arise when one person's need changes as the result of the illness. If I need more closeness because I am sick, and my partner needs more distance because they have exhausted themselves in my care, then the distance becomes hard to bridge. My need for closeness competes with my partner's need for distance. This is an example in which the patient's need competes with the need of a loved one. It requires open and honest conversation to bridge differences for partners to both feel seen and heard and work out arrangements to accommodate each other's needs, otherwise competing needs will lead to sad situations, disappointments, misunderstandings, and conflict.

Mary, a professor of literature, had many responsibilities as thesis and dissertation advisor. She loved her work and was a dedicated teacher, beloved by her mentees. When she was diagnosed with uterine cancer, one of her students asked that an early recommendation letter be kept on file. The student was concerned about what would happen in case of his professor's death.

Because of his own distress (some would call it selfishness), he was not capable of stepping back to consider his PhD advisor's predicament. He was preoccupied with his own concern, not about losing his advisor as a person but about losing the role she played in his life. These moments of self-absorption and thoughtlessness can be hurtful. I suggest that before acting on your hurt, you take a moment to reflect on the principle of competing and at times mutually exclusive needs. It can help to put both experiences into better perspective and not result in a seesaw of escalating emotions and conflict. If Mary can recognize the student as self-absorbed, she will be more realistic and not expect compassion from that particular mentee. If she wants compassion and understanding, she will need to seek it from a person who is capable of giving it.

I won't always display the algorithm picture as I hope you have internalized it by now. If you need a refresher, go back to Figure 20.

Another situation in which you might encounter competing needs is over what kind of supportive care to get. Group support is very popular and can be incredibly helpful, but I also have seen patients get quite distressed about it. You might seek out a support group in order to exchange information with others, only to encounter someone whose story evokes fear and negative thoughts. Maybe something about the other person reminds you of yourself and hits too close to home to maintain equanimity. Should you go to the group to get the information and deal with the fear or skip group and try to get the info online or from your doctor or a friend?

There can also be competing needs among group members. You might be looking for information exchange while others are looking for social interaction. If other people's motives are not immediately apparent to you, maybe we can revive the famous exercise to gain proficiency.

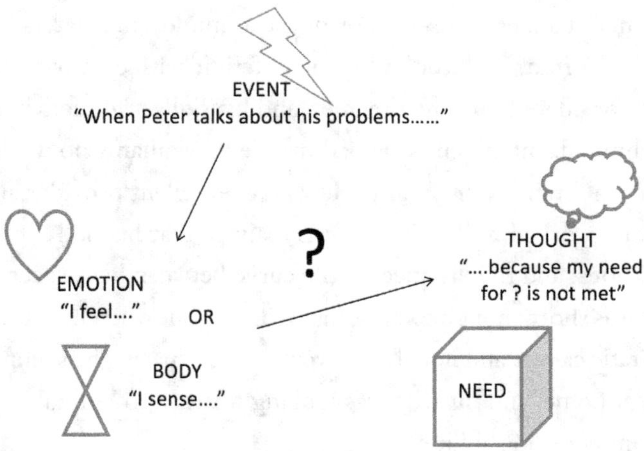

Figure 22

Maybe Peter is talkative and taking a lot of space in group. Your "when X happens, I feel" sentence might be: "When Peter talks about his problems, I feel frustrated or nervous or angry (or whatever) because my need for peace, efficiency, fairness (or whatever) is not met."

The exercise often evokes strange words that might fluster you and don't seem to make sense.

But remember that Daniel Levitin presented evidence that every conscious experience is likely stored, and David Eagleman convinced us that while most of it is not accessible, it is nonetheless influencing us. The presumably strange words that come to your mind can be very helpful in navigating your situation.

Let's assume your word was "safety," don't waste time rationalizing why you should not feel that way because you know you are safe in the group and no one is about to assault you with a butcher knife. Simply take the word seriously and encourage yourself to create a sense of safety right then and there. This could mean getting up and sneaking off to the bathroom to take a few breaths or deciding to stay and do one of the "change your feeling, change your thoughts, or change your body" exercises that I have suggested throughout the book.

Our inner changes, conscious or not, can muddy the waters. Figure 23 tells the story. A film producer had spent a lifetime with creativity. His family had always considered him the dreamer, and his skillset for activities of daily living was limited. Intelligently he had married a woman who was willing to be the practical brain of the family. He was an excellent provider and the division of roles worked well. His wife was realistic that his skill set was below her expectations, and the distance on the curve between her expectations and his skill set was short enough to not cause trouble. But when he was diagnosed with metastatic cancer and not able to work at full capacity, he spent more and more time at home, and his wife was looking forward to him taking a bigger role with family responsibilities.

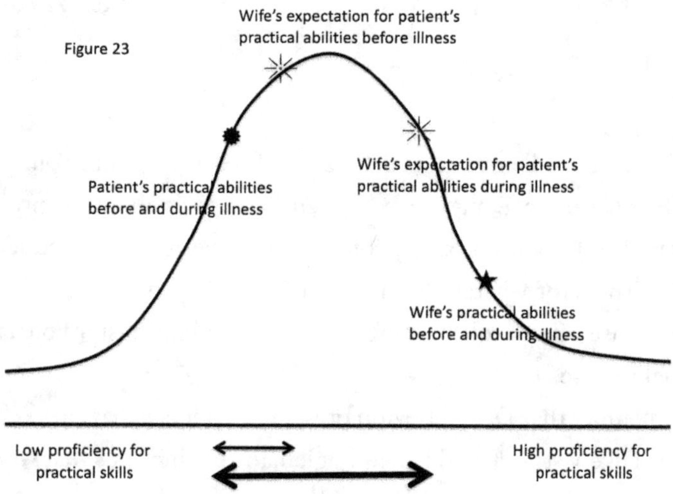

Figure 23

While her expectation was very reasonable, the film producer's skill set did not change, only his wife's expectations, and he was incapable of fulfilling it. To make matters worse, he totally withdrew and spent most of his time watching movies. She hoped for his support with the children, which she had not received enough of while he pursued his career, but instead he withdrew into the comfort of movies. Instead of the desired closeness, the river's valley became a deep ravine. Neither partner had changed their skill level. But the wife's expectation that he would use his non-existent practical skills and somehow become a more capable parent met with his augmented desire to connect to film, a medium that had always been a source of bliss and familiarity. When he was least capable of changing, his partner most needed him to change. Not surprisingly their differing needs and the increased distance on the bell curve (bold double arrow) became a constant source of conflict.

I suggest you keep competing needs in mind when interacting with your doctor, too. I frequently witness patients' interests colliding with the motivation of their doctor. I was the one who earlier claimed that patient and doctor usually share a goal of "let's get the sucker," and that is usually true, but there are some areas where their needs and desires will often collide. For starters most oncology doctors are focused on a patient's longevity. While they also consider quality of life, they cannot always understand their patients' sentiments. They get confused by patients' behavior because they do not understand the underlying motive.

When a patient refuses treatment, it does not necessarily represent a desire to die (though it could). It might be their calculation that the suffering that comes with treatment does not make it worthwhile (another illustration of a competing need). Recognizing and respecting this, the doctor might be able to make accommodations to make treatment more palatable. You can negotiate a treatment that is less debilitating, less frequent, or less aggressive. What you are willing to sign up for has to be balanced with what you can tolerate.

Physicians who get cancer will often find that they can now more easily relate to what had felt alien in their patients before. What doctors will consider exposing their patients to in terms of treatment is often not something they are willing to do themselves.

Does this mean your doctor can only really understand you when they get sick? Of course not. While there is truth to the idea that experience is a good teacher, you would not say that the only cardiologist capable of treating you is the one who has had a heart attack. As a patient, it should not be your job to educate your doctor. At the same time, please understand that while physicians have your best interest at heart, they cannot always execute perfectly because they simply cannot fully relate to what you are going through.

COMPETING NEEDS WITHIN ONESELF

Needs don't only compete between people but within them, too. Manuel loved teaching. He was a middle school teacher in a suburban town. He was diagnosed with a nasty form of blood cancer. He very much identified with being a teacher. He was passionate about his work. He was adamant that he wanted to continue working while getting treatment, but he gradually realized he could not do both. To be a good teacher competed with taking care of his health.

This resulted in a major change in his mood. He became depressed and withdrawn and pushed very hard to continue working despite having very little energy. For a few months, he was just dragging. He got up, went to work, went home, and spent the rest of the time sleeping on the sofa.

Once he was able to quit work, he blossomed. He gained some of his energy back and was even able to exercise a little bit. He started spending more time with his family again. The battle between his need to work, which was closely tied to his identity and his need to take care of his health, was finally over.

Manuel had been so attached to his identity as a teacher that it required some time and processing to prioritize taking care of his health.

You might also remember Yolanda, whom I mentioned when discussing Ellen Langer and mindset. Yolanda had a great need to help, to be helpful, and support others, but playing the role once she was in the cancer world challenged her desire for equanimity and peace. Her needs competed within Yolanda just as Manuel's identity as a teacher competed with his need to focus on his health. Once Yolanda had insight into her situation, she had more choices. She was able to fulfill her need to be helpful by volunteering at a food bank. And she also took it upon herself to work on managing her fears about her own illness and eventually experienced some peace and equanimity, even when she was exposed to other people's cancer.

Two needs I often see clash in cancer patients are quality and perfection. As a cancer patient, you want the highest quality of care, but often that gets confused with perfect care. The former is important, the latter doesn't exist. If you are unhappy with your care, ask yourself if you are, in fact, getting low-quality care, which demands a change, or is your expectation for perfection arising because your life is at stake?

The wish for perfection is fully understandable when one's life is at stake, but you will also be chronically disappointed. Mathematics comes close to perfection, not medicine. Medicine is as much an art as it is a science.

SUBJECTIVITY OF EXPERIENCE

We have seen that differing needs between different people can cause conflict and also that we can struggle with competing needs within ourselves. But when we talk about needs (again let me say that "needs" means "wants and desires," and not just absolute necessities, even though they often feel that way), we also have to consider the subjectivity of experience and perception. How I define reliability might be very different from how you define reliability. We are not just dealing with different needs but with how we each define needs.

This subjectivity is in part of why I decided to use Google definitions as a starting point. Google usually defines words in the way many of us understand them. But it would probably make the experts in the respective fields cringe because the definitions are often not terribly precise. The example of needs, wants, and desires illustrates opposite sides of the continuum, using simplicity for the sake of understanding versus using complexity for the sake of accuracy. Words and communication are subjective and relative.

We do not always start from the same place when we begin the marathon race of conversations about what things mean. Don't you sometimes find yourself in fatiguing conversations with a loved one or a friend that turn into arguments that are based in the fact that you define things differently? And to make matters worse: it is not just definitions that differ but expectations, which also exist on a continuum.

I will never forget witnessing an argument between two family members in a family that was disintegrating in the face of a cancer challenge. The fight ended with the sentence, "If you have unreasonable expectations that a normal person cannot understand, then there is something wrong with you." Wow, now that is a powerful series of judgmental statements. First, that the expectation is unreasonable! Second, that a normal person cannot understand it (Normal and abnormal in reference to what?). It implies that the person who made the request is in the wrong, when in fact there might be something wrong with the person who made the statement instead!

But we can also interpret the situation as two people simply being somewhere different on the bell curve. The expectation in fact might not have been unreasonable, just higher than the other person was able to fulfill. And rather than judging the other by saying, "I feel overwhelmed with fulfilling your request, so I decided that your request is abnormal," we might simply express feeling overwhelmed. When you watch people argue, it often ends up being a festival of trying to convince the other that you are right and they are wrong, and in fact they're just in different places on the bell curve without realizing it.

Early in **Chapter 3**, in our discussion of how we all process stressful events differently with respect to emotionality, cognition, and body experience, I mentioned that there can be differences with respect to pretty much anything as soon as two people enter the same space. These differences are crucial to consider not just when you find yourself in conflict with others but also with yourself. What is the expectation you have for yourself? Is it possible to be happy in a concentration camp? Is it possible to be happy with cancer? Please remember that your satisfaction is indirectly proportional to your expectation. The higher the expectation, the lower the satisfaction. I don't want to deter you from striving for happiness with your cancer, but let's make sure to start with tolerance and acceptance first.

INDIVIDUALS IN AN ERA OF EVIDENCE-BASED MEDICINE

In the context of our discussion about where we fit on the bell curve, I'd like to introduce the concept of "evidence-based medicine." The term suggests that we should only use treatments that were tested, preferably in large groups of people, and found beneficial for a large proportion of them. While this is a laudable goal, the reality of life is more complex. The basic idea is that we try a treatment on a group of people based on the best possible knowledge available and hope to help as many people as possible while hurting as few as possible. Image the bell curve we discussed and trying to capture the broadest possible slice that represents as many people as possible.

Sometimes it can mean treating a subset of people on the curve, which might be quite small, for example everybody with migraines. Not everybody in the population has migraines, but for those with migraines, we want to help as many as possible. "Evidence-based medicine" means making treatment recommendations that will help the largest possible group, which unfortunately also means not only that we will not treat everybody but that sometimes we might even hurt some. In other words, evidence-based medicine is a compromise. We aim to offer treatment that will be effective for as many people as possible while causing as little damage as possible.

It is very important that you understand this as a cancer patient because you will undergo treatments and you want to make sure to get the treatment with the best chance of doing good and the least chance of doing harm. There is one problem. The treatment unfortunately is not individualized for you. It was designed to help as many people on the bell curve as possible. Before you start any treatment, you have little idea of what it will do to you as an individual. Before treatment you don't know if you are going to be in the segment of the curve for whom it will be successful.

If medical decision-making is an issue you're facing right now, you can jump ahead to the respective section in **Chapter 11**. And here is a link to a YouTube presentation specifically addressing the topic of decision-making conundrum and uncertainty: (https://www.youtube.com/watch?v=PhX13NgDgxc&t=194s)

INDIVIDUALIZING TREATMENT

While I believe that evidence-based medicine is important (it's our best bet overall), I also believe that we need to strive for individualization in treatment. In some ways this is what this book is about. In the next paragraph, I want to demonstrate how important individualization is.

Most people take their breath for granted. I already emphasized its importance on well-being in **Chapter 6**. Many meditations and relaxation techniques have breath as a core feature, as it is a strong natural inducer of vagal tone (De Couck et al., 2019), and thus helps you relax. Not one session with a client goes by without me suggesting breathing deeply. As I noted earlier, I frequently interact with patients who associate breathing with some amount of distress. There are several possible causes for this negative association. Someone with asthma, for example, has scary associations with breathing from times when they could not take a breath for granted. For them the experience "breath" is associated with not having any breath, which is part of an asthma attack. Not surprisingly, with some asthma sufferers, my suggestion to breathe in a particular way is met with reluctance.

Patients with a history of trauma often have a complex relationship with breathing. During trauma people will often hold their breath as part of a freeze response. Playing dead is an evolutionary leftover of staying safe. Trauma victims can get quite unsettled when I ask them to take a breath. For them holding their breath represents safety or calmness.

Needless to say, it is very unpleasant to experience distress as part of a relaxation exercise! As a provider of advice, I have to be very thoughtful and observant. I cannot assume that breath exercises work for everybody. If you happen to be in this category, don't despair. There are other exercises in this book that achieve the same goal of helping you feel less distressed.

Guided imagery is in a similar category. Guided imagery exercises have become very popular for cancer patients, and I recommend them all the time. While it is a wonderful tool that contributes much to relaxation, it also has to be administered with exploratory caution. A common instruction in guided imagery is to "find a safe place." It is sometimes not until patients do the exercise that they realize that they have never experienced a safe place. This is particularly true of people with prior trauma. Instead of providing relaxation, a guided imagery exercise will trigger distress.

This is why I recommend, despite my full support for "evidence-based medicine," that you stay curious about your individual responses and idiosyncrasies.

Another situation in which individualization is key is in approaching meditation. The question of whether to meditate with open or closed eyes raises interesting issues. Let's explore this through an exercise.

You can do this one lying down, sitting, or even standing up. Place your hands palm down on your thighs. Take a moment to look at something that is straight ahead of you without bending your neck. Fix your eyes on whatever it is you have decided to look at.

Now take a deep breath and move your hands from your thighs to your chest or abdomen and exhale. Keep your hands on your belly or chest, so you can feel the air moving as you breathe in and out.

Take a moment to assess where to place yourself on the continuum of comfort. Do you feel comfortable or uncomfortable or something in between right now as you are listening into your body, emotions, and thoughts?

Take a few breaths while you explore your comfort level.

Next I want you to close your eyes while keeping your hand on your chest or belly and continue taking deep and slow breaths. Do you notice a difference with respect to comfort or discomfort with your eyes open versus closed?

Choose the one that facilitates comfort and decreases discomfort. If you are more comfortable meditating with your eyes open, do that. If you feel more relaxed with your eyes closed, then that's the right choice for you. Don't follow a particular instruction as part of a regimen if it does not suit you.

It is not just that the body keeps the score of bad stuff, as Bessel Van der Kolk teaches us. It is also true that the body signals us with its wisdom. The body is an important source of information. If you listen, there is much to gain.

PART III

CANCER-SPECIFIC ISSUES

While part I and II contained information that is true and useful, whether you have cancer or not, part III presents issues that arise specifically for cancer patients. I mentioned in the beginning of the book that the exercises in this book and the physiology they are based on apply to everybody, whether or not you deal with cancer. Now I am discussing these concepts more specifically through the lens of cancer. While you are reading, I always want you to keep in mind the following road map that can help you illuminate your own situation:

1) Mr. Baldwin's ping-pong with life in the face of incognito.
2) Use your thoughts, emotions, and body sensations as signals to pay attention to what might be missing.
3) Ask the question, "What do I need?" Acknowledge competing needs and hierarchy of needs.
4) There is a good chance that you experience distress, aka sympathetic hyperarousal. Are you paying attention and shifting to parasympathetic tone consistently?
5) Ask yourself where you fit on the continuum of variations of human characteristics and motivations.
6) Ask yourself whether you are minimizing self-judgment and consider the feasibility of your plans and actions.
7) Every action and every non-action has pros and cons. Ask yourself whether you are considering the cost and benefit of your choices.
8) Use your personalized action algorithm.
9) Remember that the higher the expectations, the higher the disappointment.

I will make frequent reference to previous chapters and encourage you to reread basic principles as they apply to specific cancer-related questions. It will help you consolidate some ideas and also give you an opportunity to deepen your practice. As I have emphasized many times and illustrated with studies: We learn and grow most through experience and practice.

I want to be very clear that the following chapters are not a guide of what to do about the cancer itself or its treatment. We will continue to look at cancer through the lens of distress in different phases of illness and treatment with the goal of making you more effective in dealing with your unwelcome houseguest.

CHAPTER 10.

Pre-existing Mental Health Conditions

As we discussed early on, the distress most cancer patients experience does not warrant a mental health diagnosis, at least not in numbers any greater than the rest of the population. If you encounter problems with your thinking and your emotions while dealing with cancer, they often stem from how the experience with cancer distresses your heap of cells. This does not mean there aren't people who enter the cancer process with a mental health diagnosis or walk away from cancer with one, and we have to be alert to that when it arises. But you also need not to be surprised that even if you struggled a lot emotionally prior to getting sick, you might not necessarily feel horrific during cancer. The following story illustrates this well.

Jenny had always been sensitive. Challenges easily threw her off, surprises were hard to deal with. In personal relationships, she was easily hurt, and in work relationships, she got overly self-conscious. She walked around with labels stuck to her, covering a range from "Generalized Anxiety Disorder" to "Dysthymic Disorder" to "Borderline Personality."

She was not surprised when she was diagnosed with breast cancer since she knew that she had inherited a genetic predisposition from her mother. Surprising to her and others, Jenny felt calm and composed during her treatment. She treasured the attention and support she received during treatment. She felt well taken care of. She was the center of attention. However, as soon as treatment had completed, Jenny's old symptoms reemerged. She struggled with the same issues she'd struggled with before her cancer diagnosis.

This is why I treat a mental health diagnosis in cancer care with caution. I didn't want to challenge Jenny's previous diagnosis, even though I was not sure she actually qualified for any of the labels she had received. The important point here is that Jenny felt better during treatment. That seems paradoxical. You feel better while you have cancer? But when you look, however, at Jenny's personality, it makes perfect sense. She was someone who enjoyed attention, comfort, and support, and that all came along with being sick. Furthermore, since Jenny had a family history of cancer, the diagnosis that comes as a shock to many did not shock her. Looking at Jenny from the perspective of need hierarchies, her feeling well made perfect sense.

Martin's situation prior to his cancer diagnosis was far worse than Jenny's. As a young man, he showed signs of serious mental health issues in high school. While he was able to graduate, he got emotionally lost in college and could not deal with the required independence. He became severely depressed.

For Martin the diagnosis of major depression was appropriate. He was not able to hold a job and moved back in with his mother. Like many other young people, he did not have regular health checks. When a dark spot on his back grew to a size that was big enough to catch his attention, it was too late. Martin had metastatic melanoma. He fought bravely, his depression intermittently lifting, even when the cancer spread to his brain. He had numerous treatments extending his lifespan.

One day the cancer came back yet again, this time in a tricky spot in his brain behind one eye. When he learned that the available treatment with radiation would jeopardize his vision, he called it quits. He did not want to receive any more treatments. Accepting his decision was a herculean task for his parents and his one sister. However, as soon as Martin started hospice care, his mood lifted. Like Jenny he felt well taken care of. He was not afraid to die. In fact he even expressed that leaving this earth would free him from his debilitating depression.

Most people have difficulty relating to Jenny's and Martin's stories. We need to take them seriously. If you think about the bell curve, you will understand that everybody fits somewhere on the continuum, and for some, that is at the farther ends. If you have not done so already, you will find the spot where you belong with whatever choices you make or beliefs you have. And I hope you will do so with the least judgment possible.

For both Martin and Jenny, their mental health problems prior to diagnosis did not get worse during cancer; if anything they got better. Sometimes, however, a preexisting mental health condition can make things more difficult. Researchers at Ohio State University (Shelby et al., 2008) found that women with a history of depression were twice as likely to develop posttraumatic stress after cancer; with a prior history of anxiety, it was even three times as high.

It was a small study, but the findings are consistent with my clinical experience. Being diagnosed with cancer can be the equivalent to being deployed to a war zone, particularly for those with pre-existing mental health problems. Mental health conditions in cancer patients are associated with poorer outcomes (Giese-Davis et al., 2011). Cancer patients with a psychiatric disorder report less perceived social support than their non-psychiatric peers, a perception that disappears with psychopharmacological treatment (Costa-Requena et al., 2013).

As we have discussed, a cancer diagnosis and treatment often result in an activation of a stress response, sometimes exacerbating earlier mental conditions. Effective treatment of your mental health can prove clinically challenging during a time when you feel a lack of control and want stability. You might reject a necessary change or adjustment in medication because the change symbolizes instability. If not addressed, such concerns carry the risk of jeopardizing your health. Collaboration and communication between all invested parties are crucial.

Terry, a patient with brain cancer, was adamant about not discontinuing the bupropion (best known as Wellbutrin) she had taken for depressive symptoms for years. There was only one problem. Brain cancer increases the risk for seizures, and so does bupropion. Taken together the risk increases. I have talked about competing needs. Here is a perfect example. Terry preferred the stability of a medication that had worked well for her to the trial of a different antidepressant medication, which represented uncertainty. She was willing to accept the increased risk of seizures. Similarly a gentleman with a longstanding history of bipolar disorder refused adjustments in his lithium dosage despite taking sub-therapeutic levels to "not rock the boat."

In a busy oncological setting, physicians are less likely to have the time and skill to detect the deeper meaning psychotropic medication can have to patients. Here's another example of incognito. Physicians helping to bring to the surface the patient's incognito motivation for not wanting to change the medication would help patients make a more informed decision. Patients might still choose not to change the medication, but their decision will be based not in fear but in self-knowledge and self-respect.

You can see how important it is to address mental health conditions, but I cannot emphasize strongly enough that you must not confuse symptoms of distress with mental health problems—and often you will have to be the one to help your care team recognize this, too.

Having read **Chapter 6**, you should be a pro at recognizing symptoms of distress. Unfortunately many patients, family, friends, *and* professionals, confused and distressed by natural changes in emotions and thoughts, tend to identify them as mental health disorders. Careful assessment will both hasten getting you help early and efficiently, if you need it, and avoid imposing diagnoses on patients without prior psychiatric conditions who are experiencing distress. If you are a healthcare provider, I encourage you to use psychiatric diagnosis with caution in cancer patients. While it is important to not miss any, it is as important to not incorrectly diagnose them either. Recall **Chapter 9** and remind yourself to evaluate people on a curve and assess if they are within "normal." It decreases the chance that you will miscategorize the patients.

Once again it's all a matter of degree. Depending on where you fall on the continuum, some approaches mentioned here might not be suitable. When I work with patients with severe mental health conditions, I am torn about using some of the exercises described in this book. Thinking can get so thwarted and rigid that suggesting positive thinking while standing on one leg can feel offensive. Fortunately, when I am off base in my assessment, I can see it immediately in how my patients respond and let their response guide my choices. The same way Jenny's experience helps us remember the "needs principle" during cancer, both Terry's and the gentleman with bipolar disorder's experiences illustrate not only the importance of recognizing your needs but also of the "continuum principle," which emphasizes that we need to address individual differences, even if they don't make sense at first glance.

And it is worth taking the risk for the occasional gaffe. Because for every missed mental health diagnosis in cancer patients, there are even more patients on the other side of the continuum who gratefully exclaim, "I am so glad I am not crazy" when I explain the context of mind and body in distress and how feeling upset, having your thoughts jumbled, or your emotions flow can mimic "crazy."

Fortunately more and more hospitals are screening cancer patients for distress and looking at spiritual, emotional, practical, and physical needs. Unfortunately there are still inadequate services to address them and never enough money to support them.

CHAPTER 11

Dealing with Diagnosis

SHOCK OF DIAGNOSIS

With cancer and other serious illnesses, there is that one particular moment when life changes permanently. When patients first receive the news about their cancer, they are almost always surprised and shocked. Sometimes the delivery itself is shocking. You might be about to sit down to dinner when the phone rings. "I have what? How can this be?" Your family is staring at you in shock while you are trying to sit down to process the news. Or maybe you were peacefully riding in your car whistling to the sound of the music on the radio when the phone rang. "I cannot cure you" is the first sentence you hear. Dazed, you pull over, sweating, stunned.

These responses are common, particularly if you had little adversity prior to getting ill. Some patients describe the feeling as "falling off a cliff," some will even tell their doctors, "You cannot drop me off a cliff like that." We saw in **Chapter 8**, from the study by Campbell and colleagues, that distress about diagnosis is among the top ten unmet needs. Having a strong emotional reaction is not an indication of mental illness!

Unfortunately poor delivery of the challenging news is often part of the shock. It is a reasonable expectation not wanting to hear it on the phone or receive the devastating news by email. You also should not have to wait for a meeting with the doctor after the diagnostic process of bloodwork and scans to discussing the results. In reality there's much room to grow on that front.

Let's revisit Figure 9 to gain insight how the diagnosis affected you or how it affects you now, if you were recently diagnosed. You saw this image in **Chapter 8** when we discussed needs and have hopefully integrated the exercise into other aspects of your life as I encouraged in that chapter.

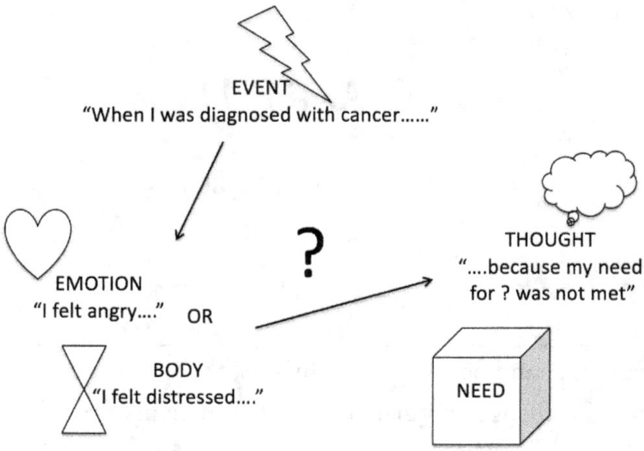

Figure 9

Figure 10 is the practice version of what you just saw, with some assisting options I will walk you through to help you become a solo flyer. The exercise will give you some perspective about yourself rather than the sheer horror of the diagnosis. The exercise would look something like this:

Start by identifying your emotion and/or body sensations, which leads up to defining the need. If options look familiar, circle them; otherwise add your own. If you struggle, you can always refer to the emotions and needs inventory in the respective **Chapters 5** and **8**. The following practice sentence will sound familiar from **Chapter 8** when we discussed needs. "When I was diagnosed with cancer, I felt angry (for more emotionally oriented people) or distressed (for more physically oriented people) because my need for (blank) was not met."

And before you start practicing, I want to reiterate an important distinction about physical symptoms and sensations. I discussed this in the section on **Ego Congruency** in **Chapter 7,** but it is so important for most cancer patients that I cannot mention it often enough. Recall Jordan, who wondered what the cause of his belly pain was. It took him a while to differentiate tumor discomfort from distress-related discomfort. As you probably know from your own body and experience, it is not always easy to know the difference. Not knowing if your symptoms are related to distress or to the tumor pressing on nerves or bones or organs is disconcerting and confusing and evokes fear.

Cancer comes with so many physical symptoms, and the treatment comes with so many physical side effects, that I don't want you to conclude easily that your symptoms are stress based. But while the distinction is difficult, it is worthwhile to consider the activation of the autonomic nervous system as a possible cause. You cannot do harm by decreasing your distress and seeing what happens to your symptoms. If you learn that they are caused by the tumor, then you have a at least a clearer brain to solve the problem.

The data in Figure 10 suggest that the unmet needs in this example could have been certainty, safety, control, support, and independence. When you do the exercise, don't just consider these examples, but let the word emerge "incognito" style. This part is important because it is a more effective way to get to the 99 percent of motivations that happen outside of our awareness. If you forgot what "incognito" refers to, you can consolidate by rereading the section on **Incognito** in **Chapter 3**.

Figure 10

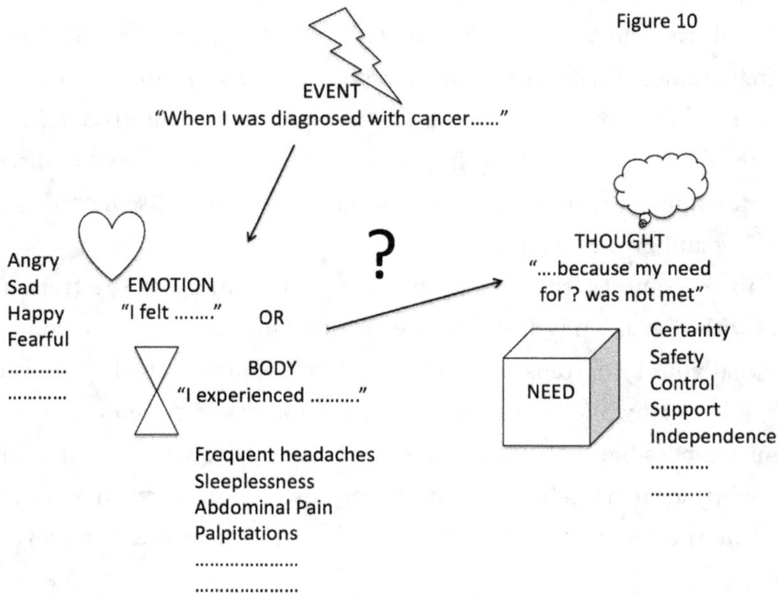

Again, if you are a patient who was recently diagnosed, take a moment to walk yourself through the exercise and discover what core needs were not met at the time of diagnosis. If your diagnosis is in the past, as is likely if you are reading this book, you can mentally place yourself back into the situation and still do the exercise also. The discoveries you make can help you better handle future stressors.

While you are always welcome to walk yourself through all steps, you can also skip "emotion" and "body" and go straight to, "When I was diagnosed with cancer, my need for 'x' was not met." While that is simpler and faster, some people enjoy going through their emotional and physical experiences to let the word emerge.

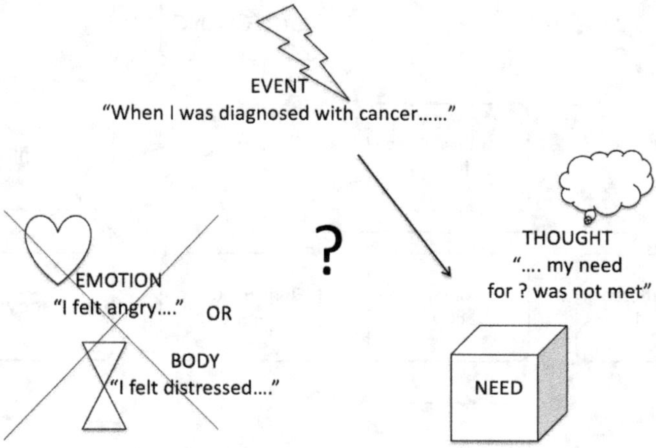

Figure 11

Whatever words come up in the exercise are an important source of information about yourself and are useful to tap into what makes you tick. The words represent important needs and motivations and serve as a guide to take action.

In **Chapter 8**, I took you through the practice when the word was *control*, and in **Chapter 9**, you briefly considered *caregiving* in Figure 20. Let's expand your exploration with this need. Imagine you are a cancer patient who at your core is a caregiver. When you cannot fulfill that need for caregiving because you're sick, you will be in for a tough ride. Look at Figure 20 again as I walk you through your options.

Figure 20

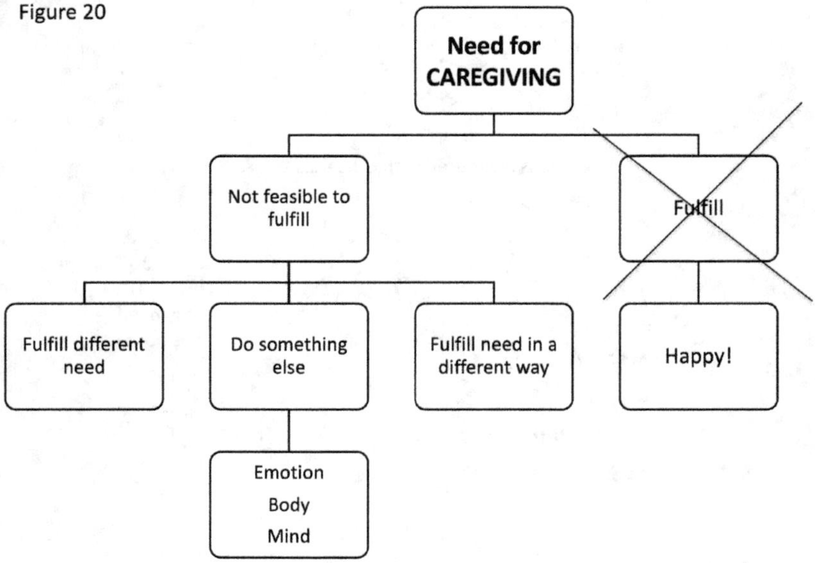

If caregiving is at the center of who you are, you may have a strong reaction to not being able to do it while you are experiencing your cancer, but you might be able to fulfill the need in a different way. Maybe you are too weak and fatigued to take care of someone else, but you can become the designated caretaker of your houseplants. And if that does not sound appealing you, try fulfilling a different need. Perhaps you received valuable support during your ordeal. You can channel your desire to give care by expressing gratitude and thanks to the people who helped you.

If you want something more mundane, organizational tasks can help, like sorting closets or doing dishes. Whatever needs you have can be redirected onto a different object, or you can transform the need into a different one.

Many people need help with this idea of what's reasonable or feasible for them. They'll come up with fantastic alternative ideas, but they are not realistic, and their expectations of themselves are not based in the reality of the situation, and that in itself will be a source of frustration. The body can, however, be appeased by fulfilling any need-based activity. It does not have to be cancer related.

When I propose this, people often discover that they had already started an activity that resembled a core need without realizing the transposition. As

I described earlier, humans under duress tend to intensify a to-them familiar coping strategy. In the caregiving example, there is a good chance you will struggle with not being able to give care while undergoing cancer treatment and wonder why you started planting perennials on your balcony. These unconsciously chosen replacement activities are puzzling until you see their purpose.

Once you realize that the behavior is motivated to satisfy a particular need, you can choose to satisfy the need or to learn to live without it. And if nothing works, you can always turn to the mini-exercises that are spread throughout the book to soothe your emotions, calm your body, and relax your mind, which in Figure 20 is labeled as to do something else.

CAUSALITY OF DIAGNOSIS

It is not at all uncommon for people to think they have caused their cancer. The thought can haunt you from the time of diagnosis to the end of treatment and beyond. You might also feel betrayed by your body. You trusted your heap of cells until you didn't. Or you assign fault to yourself for getting sick, at times being haunted by feelings of guilt, even when your illness is not related to prior behavior. These are examples in which the need for understanding can be quite confusing.

These thoughts can be very stressful, even if the doctor assures you that there is no connection between your behavior and your cancer. "If I did not cause the cancer, what did?" is usually the very next question. We want to know.

People are very imaginative with respect to finding presumed causes for their cancer. They attribute lifestyle choices, like diet, exercise, and stress, to the development of cancer. Sometimes people will attribute a very specific event as the cause of their illness. Karen, a devout Catholic, was convinced that an abortion earlier in life was the cause of her multiple myeloma subbing as a punishment. You'll read more about Karen in **Chapter 15** on **Religion and Spirituality**.

The derailment of regular cells into cancer, however, is a very complex process and the longing for understanding will rarely get satisfied. As a physician, I thought I was up to date on cancer development, but reading an article about it, I had to admit that my view was simplistic, antiquated, and mostly wrong (Dushek, 2016).

Why do we humans rush to fill the unknown with a presumed cause? Because not knowing is super stressful. I believe we find the answer in the "need principle." Humans are not good at uncertainty. In order to satisfy the desire to understand, we would rather fill in the blank of "why" with something that makes sense to us, even if it is incorrect than tolerate uncertainty. Remember Daniel Levitin who taught us in **Chapter 4** on **Thinking** that the right brain is the fact tracker and the left brain is responsible for "making order out of chaos, for making sense of things in the world that don't always add up." The only problem is that the left brain makes stuff up and lies to suit the purpose of making sense, even if you misattribute a wrong cause to your illness.

Understanding also gives us a sense of control to change. If you are convinced that it was the sugar cookies you overindulged in that led to your cancer, then you believe that you can do something beneficial by stopping eating cookies. Going all organic and antioxidant will not just presumably help you get healthy, it is also an attempt at rectifying an assumed mistake. But all of these ideas are ultimately just ideas, rarely based in the reality of your body.

While we can all optimize our health by improving our behavior, I do not want you to add distress by trying to fill uncertainty with a fictional sense of certainty.

People will also wonder if prior life experiences might have caused stress and then, as trapped emotions, might have caused their cancer. They wonder if work stress might have contributed to the development of their illness. Hear me please. It is always a good idea to decrease distress (in many ways that is what this book is all about), but assigning causality is *very tricky business*.

I am well-aware that there is literature that associates stress with the development and progression of cancer. I am willing to discuss that possibility, and there is some science that supports it, but speculation itself causes distress. As long as you realize that the purpose of understanding is to help you do things better and as best you can, I am all for it, but if making the association is an attempt at regaining the illusion of safety and control, I urge you to do what you can to avoid this type of thinking.

The idea that we can be distressed about stress is a common topic I debate with cancer patients. It is my clinical experience that it will be easier to change your body state, e.g. slow your heart rate, if you utilize the algorithm of taking action and go down the path of "doing something else" than it is to change your thinking from "my work stress caused my cancer" to "I don't know what caused my cancer." But ultimately you have to explore how the algorithm works best for you.

The ultimate message is this: pick whatever works to help you not distort your thoughts and dampen your emotion through chronic sympathetic hyperarousal.

If you are not in the mood for the algorithm exercise, you might yank out your parasympathetic exercise list from **Chapter 6** on **Body**. The bottom line: If you want to improve your health, creating fictitious reality to battle your inability to tolerate uncertainty is not the most efficient way.

Of course not being able to identify a "cause" is often distressing, too. Elizabeth still remembers the sudden shift in experience when being told the news about her illness. She described needing an understanding on how "her body could have let her down" since she had always taken good care of it. While her body had always been a friendly ally, it suddenly became a disappointing enemy.

"I always had such a good relationship with my body, and now I have to find peace with a twin sister who let me down."

Fortunately this patient was able—after a brief obsession with mortality—to refocus her attention on what is relevant in her current life. Fairness and justice are human desires. Cancer cannot fulfill that need. Cancer is neither fair nor just.

The process of finding peace with your diagnosis becomes even more complex if you did engage in behavior that might have caused or at least contributed to the development of cancer. Patients who smoke or down a pint of whiskey a day, for example, will find themselves in that category. I cannot use the explanation of the complexity of cancer cell development because in those circumstances there is a high chance there is a correlation between their behavior and their cancer.

In such cases the process of finding equanimity is about finding peace with having messed up. Even though you will never know whether your unhealthy behavior contributed, it is more effective to find peace with having messed up than talking yourself into not knowing.

If you are haunted by thoughts about causality and the guilt that's associated with it, you can pick any of the exercises in this book that decrease negative thought content, shift emotion, or learn to tolerate non-perfection.

What all these examples have in common is the difficulty of dealing with statistical probabilities. By now you are a pro at probabilities and normal distributions (or at the very least you have reached conscious incompetence!). And you can go back to **Chapter 9** if you need a refresher. Yes, smoking increases the risk of certain cancers and so does drinking a daily pint of liquor. But you can get those cancers, even if you haven't smoked or abused alcohol. And you can get cancer if you have lived a perfectly healthy life.

Despite my encouragement to use the algorithm generously to find anything to make you feel better, I also encourage you to find a gentle way to learn to live with not knowing. Mixing the topic of statistical probabilities with the topic of human needs wastes a lot of energy. Understandable use of energy but usually not useful. We will discuss this again later in this chapter in the section on medical decision-making.

Even a "bad" action, such as smoking, does not necessarily lead to a bad outcome. In fact 90 percent of smokers will not get lung cancer. I certainly don't want you to take this as an encouragement to smoke since it is also true that roughly 90 percent of lung cancer patients did smoke, and even though "only" 10 percent of smokers get lung cancer, the American Cancer Society estimates that just in 2022 alone, 236,740 people will be diagnosed with lung cancer and about 130,180 will die. That is a lot of people. It is still a "no brainer" not to smoke because the logic "I have a 9/10 chance that it will not affect me," does not make a good argument. 213,068 smokers are the 10 percent of smokers who most likely did get sick from smoking.

(Don't be surprised that the number is smaller than the total yearly number since I had to subtract the 10 percent non-smokers who get lung cancer despite never having smoked a cigarette). The point I want you to remember is that statistics *never* describe an individual. That's what makes statistics so challenging and at times confusing and stressful. You never know whether or not the numbers will apply to you.

FINDING PEACE WITH THE DIAGNOSTIC PROCESS

Getting diagnosed can take a while. Geoffrey was a young, carefree nineteen-year-old. He did not think much about the lesion on the side of his tongue. His dentist and his primary care doctor did not either. When the lesion did not heal, the wheels of medicine were set in motion. A surgeon tried a skin flap, a psychiatrist an antidepressant for tongue biting. Nothing helped. No one thought of cancer until it was too late. Geoffrey died from tongue cancer short of his 21st birthday. Of course most stories do not have a sad and deadly outcome like this one, but understandably some lead to anger and disappointment in the diagnostic process. If Geoffrey's doctors had recognized the cancer and taken action sooner, mightn't he still be alive? Maybe but…

A number of different symptoms lead people to their first visits with the primary care doctor. What usually follows is a journey from specialist to specialist until the dreaded word "cancer" enters the room. It is easy to feel convinced that it was the doctor's fault that you weren't diagnosed earlier. We immediately second guess that the prognosis might have been better "if we had caught it earlier." In Geoffrey's case, it was a tragic combination of constellations that no one generated the thought until it was too late that "young person" and "tongue cancer" belong in the same sentence. Every player in the diagnostic process was biased because of Geoffrey's young age. A statistically unlikely scenario has a much smaller chance at getting caught than an obvious one. But for the person experiencing a late diagnosis, it is never easy.

Statistics are never clear-cut with respect to the individual. Are we going to biopsy a bump on the neck if we have a history of breast cancer? Chances are the bump is benign, but if you are the person who finds herself with a metastatic recurrence after the biopsy, finding peace will be a challenge.

We learned earlier that patients experience anger and guilt about certain behaviors. In the diagnostic process, the anger is often directed at the doctor but also at oneself or both. You might have sensed that you were sick but chose not to seek an evaluation. You will never know if an earlier diagnosis would have had a better outcome, but emotionally you will experience guilt and wonder if the timing of the diagnosis was also your responsibility. Sometimes it is not the diagnosis itself but the form of delivery. A patient reported an efficient diagnostic process but being shocked by the delivery of bad news over the phone rather than in person.

Often feelings of regret and anger or sadness dissipate once treatment starts, but doubts about whether the outcome would have been better often linger and sometimes remain. "We are where we are, and let's move forward" is often not the best way to solve this emotional conundrum. When your life is on the line to find peace does not always follow the logic of reasoning. Exercises to "accept" are not my first line treatment because they often go against the patient's sentiment, but I suggest to patients to assess what percentage of their thought content is being consumed by negative thinking about the diagnostic process. If it is high, I recommend minimizing the thought content by the various exercises you now have available and remember the algorithmic process that accompanied you in Figure 12 through 15. When the brain is busy with something else, it cannot ruminate as you learned in **Chapter 4** on **Thinking**. If thoughts still dominate finding peace often has to do with acceptance and forgiveness of presumed error. When your life is at stake, that is a lot to ask for but not impossible to achieve. This is where I often resort to my "needs approach." If we can't find peace with the injustice and imperfection, can we re-direct our attention towards needs that we can feasibly satisfy?

DIAGNOSTIC AND THERAPEUTIC PRIORITIES

You heard about Manuel earlier. He is the dedicated teacher who had a shift in focus and priorities after he became ill, and his illness taught him to say "no" more easily. Four years into being sick, he shared how important it would have been to him if at the time of diagnosis doctors would not have just focused on treating his cancer. His illness made his bones brittle, and a bone in his spine gradually collapsed not unlike what can happen in people who have osteoporosis. Manuel could not stand tall anymore, something he had always prided himself in. It also limited his ability to exercise. He expressed that he would have appreciated having been informed about that possibility at the time of diagnosis. Not wanting to defend the lack of communication, I also understand how it happened.

When your health team is doing everything in its power to fight for your life, they can tend to forget about other parts of your health and well-being. This is not only true at the time of diagnosis but after treatment as well, something we will look at in the survivorship section. This is a sad illustration of prioritizing needs. In the heat of the need "survival," the need "health maintenance" might not make the cut.

If you have the resources, hiring a health advocate can help. They can take a neutral and complete view of your situation and make sure that nothing falls through the cracks. As a patient, you simply cannot; you should not expect yourself to fulfill this task on your own. Sometimes, unfortunately, we have to walk ourselves through the "algorithm" of options if some needs cannot be met.

DEALING WITH THE WORLD AROUND YOU

Privacy

The need for privacy differs from person to person. Remember our discussion of normal distribution in **Chapter 9**. Now I want you to do a self-assessment of your need for privacy and place yourself on the bell curve. Are you someone who only will tell a few trusted friends, or are you someone who posts your diagnosis on Facebook? This is fundamental as I see a lot of disappointment from the lack of recognition of differences in need of privacy. If you are more private than the majority of people you know, you have to be thoughtful about what to share.

If you revisit the section on **Normal distribution and the Bell Curve** in **Chapter 9**, you might recall the possibility of being in the minority. Wanting privacy you might expect everyone else to have similar expectations and standards. Sharing your story, however, comes with a high probability that it will be shared with others by the person you shared it with. People in general mean well and want to help, but some are also curious and gossipy. If you don't want your story circulated on the playground of your children's school, be selective about sharing.

How to navigate your need for privacy while still creating a supportive network can be very challenging. What you need and what your caregivers and supportive systems need can differ drastically. Patients frequently express a need for privacy. The reason is not that they are particularly secretive, but limited energy and an overtaxed schedule force patients to optimize their time and energy. Keeping the illness private allows you to maintain a sense of normality, but it also comes at the price of not having access to all the help that could become available when sharing your illness with a bigger group of people. This is an example in which your needs might not just compete, they might in fact be mutually exclusive.

Your need for privacy is likely to change over the course of your illness as well. Maybe you were someone who was open and talkative before your diagnosis and have become more introverted and privacy-oriented since. Once again visualize the bell curve you encountered in **Chapter 9** and place yourself on the continuum with respect to your need for privacy before cancer and with cancer. If it has changed, you might have to make adjustments. You might have competing needs with others but also within yourself as well. And you might remember that the long distance on that curve comes with trouble, particularly if the distance develops suddenly with a sudden change in needs. That's why I keep reminding you to use the many exercises you have practiced as part of reading this book that can help you get through it. The basic algorithm presented in variations in Figures 12 to 15 is an image that you can carry in your head as much as you can carry one of Mr. Baldwin.

Other People's Responses

I will talk about this again in **Chapter 14** on **Caregivers Unite**, but a common desire of patients is feeling heard, understood, or supported. When you share not only the facts of what is happening to you but how you feel about it, the responses unfortunately cover the whole range from assuring you that you don't feel the way you actually feel or acknowledging that you do feel the way you feel, but that it is not a big deal to feel that way, or—even when acknowledging that what you're feeling is a big deal—being consoled that things will be better soon.

These responses to how you feel are unhelpful and are often accompanied by actions of wanting to help but being unhelpful. The source of distress from this is considerable for you as well as the people around you. And as I have emphasized many times, particularly in **Chapter 9** in the section on **Competing Needs**, the distress can be alleviated by remembering and practicing the principle of competing or exclusive needs.

When the desire to be helpful is paired with actual helplessness, the outcome for you as a patient is challenging. Awareness of the dynamic can alleviate some of the distress. This is ultimately another way of saying suck it up when you feel unheard and unsupported but also encouragement to naturally gravitate towards people and situations that are capable of giving you what you need rather than banging your head against the wall of people who can't.

What to Tell Your Children

If you have children, what you choose to tell them and not tell them and when will depend on different factors. You will find all kind of recommendations covering a broad spectrum of options. Whatever you choose, keep a few thoughts in mind. With younger children, I generally recommend less sharing over more, particularly if your cancer is the type that is likely to be curable. Children have few desires beyond normality, routine, and fitting in. The younger children are, the less they have a concept of abstraction. They don't understand the word *cancer* or its implication in your body.

If you do share about your illness, and sometimes you will have to regardless, use analogies they can relate to. Describe an illness they themselves have experienced, such as a harmless flu. It will it make it easier for them to relate to what you are going through because they do understand what *they* went through, when they were so achy and sleepy that they had to stay in bed all day.

If you choose to be open with your children or other parents or educators in school, realize that you will lose control over the flow of information. Again people generally have good intentions and want to help. There are also some who are big sharers. I have had patients describe how their children heard about another child's parent or grandparent dying of cancer and become convinced, no matter what the patient tells them, that this is what's going to happen to their mom or dad.

The human mind is quick to categorize, but as a result, it often miscategorizes. Your young child will not understand that your curable stage I cancer is different from the one that killed a classmate's grandma. This can cause much unnecessary distress. This is why I say that with young children, it can be better to withhold details.

As usual the devil is in the details. As long as you can maintain normality, keep the details to a minimum. I don't, however, want you to hear this to mean you should tiptoe around and whisper in hushed tones. Or lie and tell them you have the flu when you've lost your hair to chemotherapy.

Children are very, very perceptive. It ultimately depends on how much privacy you need and how much control you want to have over the flow of information. As usual the task is to calibrate competing needs and individualize them for your personal situation.

MEDICAL DECISION MAKING

Assembling a Team

Before you can decide what to do, you need a good treatment team. To get a treatment team together is not easy. If you think of yourself on the bell curve, you have to assess several things. If you're someone who enjoys researching, you'll need to assess if you can tolerate the distress that can be associated with researching cancer. You might want to delegate this task. Reading mortality and outcome statistics of how many people are still alive after five years is not fun. Many people do not know too much about the statistics of their illness and just get through treatment and reevaluate their situation scan to scan. Doing or not doing your own research: either one is fine.

Before deciding place yourself on the bell curve with respect to your desire to seek out your own information. If you don't think you'll be able to bear in mind that statistics do not say anything about you individually, I urge you to delegate the task to someone else, preferably someone whose judgment you really trust, because the statistics are very likely to cause you distress.

Anne had to deal with this difficult question of how much to research information yourself. She was diagnosed with a rare form of breast cancer at a young age. She was not satisfied with the information she received from her treating team, and being scientifically minded, she dived into the available medical literature on her own. To her shock, she discovered that her five-year chance of survival was less than 50 percent, and she was terrified for her two young children. She is still alive five years later, and her children are thriving, but ask yourself what you would've done if you'd been in her shoes. Research the situation and deal with the distress of the statistics or surrender to the bliss of ignorance and focus solely on staying or getting healthy?

Communicate With Your Care Team

I have emphasized the importance of communication throughout the book, but there is probably no place it matters more than with your treatment team. You want to work with people with sophisticated communication skills—and to have such skills yourself. Communication is not just about how physicians or health personnel communicate with you. It is also about how you communicate with them.

Daisy wanted to get a second opinion from a physician she believed had expertise specific to her situation, but she also did not want to annoy the physician she had already been working with. She was concerned that her need for information would jeopardize her relationship with her doctor and affect her care. Fortunately her physician was open to a collaborative approach. He appreciated that Daisy was upfront about it and readily helped facilitate the process.

It helped that she opened the discussion with him by saying that what she was going to ask was not a reflection of her unhappiness with him but an attempt at calming herself with as much information as possible. Daisy was smart enough to know that doctors, too, can feel insecure, and she preempted that outcome with her skillful use of language. Stating the motivation for your behavior—in this case, asking for a second opinion—helps prevent misinterpretation on side of the doctor. In an ideal world, you should not have to consider that doctors have needs and insecurities also, but they do.

Managing the Conundrum of Decision Making

As soon as patients receive a diagnosis, a majority go right into "getting the best treatment" mode. This is incredibly stressful as there is often no perfect or clear solution to the problem, no "best." "Be quick, but don't hurry," the famous quote of basketball coach John Wooden sums up the issue. You want to act swiftly but not rashly. But that is easier said than done when you look at the complexity of decision-making when it comes to approaching cancer.

An article by Ann Killion in the *San Francisco Chronicle* (March 20, 2019) about Nathan Adrian, a collegiate swimmer from UC Berkeley who was diagnosed with testicular cancer in 2019, described the problem perfectly. "A public-health major at Cal, Adrian found himself suddenly putting his degree to use, understanding the reports he was reading and weighing his treatment options. But as a world-class athlete, used to specific goals and success measured with a stopwatch, the gray area of statistics and probabilities surrounding cancer diagnoses could be frustrating." Decision-making, as he was learning, was not black and white but included a lot of gray.

Table 4 illustrates one of these issues from the perspective of a cost-benefit analysis.

	Outcome successful	Outcome unsuccessful
Procedure Yes	80%	20%
Procedure No	20%	80%

Imagine taking an action that works out 80 percent of the time, or four times out of five. Those are pretty good odds. A successful outcome, e.g., would be a cure. You are doing a procedure, like surgery or radiation, and a cure is a successful outcome. If you have an 80 percent chance of something working, you have to further determine what "unsuccessful" means. Does it mean simply not working, like the procedure is not successful, or is the procedure in fact working but carries potentially any harm? This is what Table 5 shows:

	Outcome successful	Outcome unsuccessful
Procedure Yes	80%	20%
Procedure No	20%	80%

CHRONIC PAIN

Looking at the numbers, you still have an 80 percent chance of success, but the box in the middle shows that there is a side effect associated with the procedure, in this case chronic pain. Would you do a procedure that has an 80 percent chance of curing you but a 50 percent chance of living with chronic pain after the procedure? Imagine you do the procedure and are among the unlucky 20 percent that don't get cured but still have a 50 percent chance of living with pain? These are incredibly difficult decisions you face every time you step in a doctor's office to discuss your choices.

If you assess any procedure, you have to contemplate risk. This is a crucial distinction of different versions of "unsuccessful" because if you choose to do a procedure, not only is there a chance that it will be unsuccessful (e.g. you might not be cured), it might be successful but have side effects, or even worse, be unsuccessful but still have side effects.

And there is a wide range of risks. Imagine the procedure carries a 10 percent risk of death. A 10 percent chance of a headache is one thing, but imagine the burden on your decision if what you are about to decide has a 10 percent chance of killing you.

Making those risk assessments is incredibly difficult. What is a reasonable risk? Often you cannot anticipate what it will mean to live with neuropathy or chronic fatigue or ringing in your ears until you experience it.

In real life, the situation is not always that extreme and always about death. Let's look at an example that illustrates the difficulty of medical decision-making (and communication and conduct as well).

Ellen was no stranger to cancer. She had experienced breast cancer a few years earlier, but a lumpectomy and radiation had taken care of it. Some years later, Ellen was diagnosed again, this time with a more advanced breast cancer. She had a mastectomy, and it was recommended that she take a medication that would reduce estrogen, a natural hormone that we all produce but that some cancer cells also thrive on. The idea was to pull all available levers to decrease the likelihood of the cancer coming back.

What happened next surprised me. Ellen is a good historian, so I don't doubt she told me the truth, but the doctor in me could not quite grasp that the exchange could have taken place in a physician's office. I am proud to be a physician and I want all doctors to be diligent and competent.

Ellen reported that her doctor said she could not provide a risk assessment specific to Ellen's situation but believed the risk of recurrence to be quite low. She refused to provide Ellen with scientific literature relevant to her situation, arguing that journal articles are written for doctors, and Ellen couldn't possibly understand them. The doctor urged Ellen to take the medicine, arguing that only about 10 percent of patients experienced side effects (shown in the box in Table 6 below) and assuring Ellen that she could always stop taking the medication if the side effects were intolerable.

The doctor pressed on, telling Ellen that patients who did not take the medicine had a 65 percent chance of recurrence whereas patients who took the medicine had only a 35 percent chance. To the doctor, the choice seemed obvious.

She did not understand why Ellen would be reluctant to take a medication that could cure her. Ellen was all ears when she heard the word "cure." To clarify she specifically asked if the doctor was saying that taking the medicine would cure her, and the answer was yes. There is a difference between the question “Will it cure me?” and “Does it have a chance at curing me?”

There are so many problems with this situation and the communication that transpired that I want to dissect it in detail. The table for Ellen’s situation looks like this:

	Cancer stays away	Cancer comes back
Take medication	65%	35%
Don’t take medication	35%	65%

(Take medication row, spanning both columns:)
Joint Pain
Hot flashes
Insomnia

If I had been the patient in this situation, I would have left the office utterly confused. First, I would have been offended that the doctor was not willing to provide me with the scientific literature. Let me be the judge of whether I can understand it. I would understand if the doctor didn’t have the time to provide me with a printed copy, but at least give me the reference, so I can dig it up myself. An informed patient is a good thing! But truly confusing is the risk assessment the doctor provided. The statement, “taking the medication will cure you,” is simply incompatible with the statement “taking the medicine results in the cancer not coming back in 65 percent of people.” A cure means that there is a 100 percent chance of the cancer not returning. So which one was it? Did taking the medication mean 65 percent chance of the cancer not returning or 100 percent?

Unfortunately I know the answer, even though I was not a fly on the wall listening into the conversation. Very little in life is 100 percent guaranteed, except for death, so I assume the 65 percent was the more likely scenario, but Ellen was so turned off by the interaction that she decided not to return.

She originally wanted the doctor's support to make a decision about medication since she was worried that the side effects of joint pain, hot flashes, and difficulty sleeping might be lasting, but that issue was never addressed. Instead Ellen opted to take her chances on the left lower quadrant box. Don't take medication, don't have side effects, but take the risk that 2/3 people in her situation will have their cancer return.

If she had chosen to take the medication, she could have been one of the women who had the effect of the medication with little or no side effects of joint pain, hot flashes, and insomnia. Or she could have taken the medicine for a trial period and reduce or stop it if the side effects had become too uncomfortable. But given what had transpired in the process of decision-making, she never took that chance.

Misinterpretation of statistical data can also have tragic consequences. Giselle had a form of blood cancer that people can live with for many years without intervention. The median life span without doing anything was ten years. Median defines the time after which 50 percent of people are still alive. At age seventy, it would have been a reasonable personal choice for Giselle to wait and see. Giselle was also informed that a stem cell transplant could cure her. What she unfortunately did not consider in her decision-making was that the procedure had a risk of death for 10 percent of people. One out of ten people die. Sadly Giselle was the one out of ten people. Even though she had a good chance of living for at least a few years without doing anything, she took the 10 percent chance of death to get cured and paid the highest price.

I had mentioned the emotional burden that comes with making a decision that carries a 10 percent risk of death. Maybe Giselle did not misinterpret the data, maybe she simply didn't hear it because she connected to the hope of a cure. Another form of confirmation bias. We unfortunately sometimes only hear what we want to hear.

Giselle's family was left with a sense that the doctors had killed their beloved mother and wife when in fact the hope of a cure was so tempting that Giselle lost sight of the risk of death. Always look at the cost and benefits and pros and cons. If you play the lottery, you have a chance at winning, albeit a small one, but the cost is a $5 ticket. In medicine a choice might feel like winning the lottery when it aims at cure, but the price can be painfully high and not just $5 for a ticket.

You might have noticed that this section on medical decision-making and statistics is sizable. I emphasize it because I see many people struggle in this area and sometimes make decisions they later regret.

When I work with patients and families, we always discuss that we need to learn to both be comfortable with a scenario happening and with it not happening. When you look at the medical decision box, there are always four possibilities:

- I can take an action, and something will happen or it will not
- I can NOT take that same action, and something will happen or it will not.

From an emotional perspective, this is very challenging. We have to make decisions based on not knowing.

Let's look at it in more detail and go back to Ellen's example. But now we will also look at the situation from an emotional perspective and not just a medical one.

If Ellen decides to take the medication, she puts herself in the group of people in which two-thirds will not get cancer again, and the only downside is that she might have to live with some side effects. If the side effects are tolerable, Ellen probably will be content.

Now imagine Ellen takes the medicine, but she has disabling side effects and the cancer comes back anyway, which it will in 1/3 people, even if they take the medication (right upper quadrant in Table 6). She will be very unhappy.

Ellen chose not to take the medicine, which meant no side effects but also living with a 65 percent risk of a cancer recurrence (left lower quadrant in Table 6). Ellen needed to be at peace with that possibility. Patients who choose this scenario often feel anticipatory guilt. "If the cancer comes back, it is my fault because I did not take the medicine." The choice can be extremely stressful.

As I'm writing this, I have to concentrate to keep the complex options presented in Table 6 straight. Remember you have to make these decisions with the distress of cancer weighing you down! Sometimes your choice will not have the best possible outcome, despite you having given it your best. Try to manage your distress as much as possible before you make decisions to optimize your decision-making ability. And if by the (un)luck of the draw you don't have the outcome you wished for, please try to not blame yourself for it.

Sometimes patients try several medicines in order to decrease their risk of recurrence. However, the side effects can be so challenging and taxing that after several tries, patients decide to stop taking the medicine.

I vividly remember Joni, a lawyer who struggled through several months of joint pain, difficulty sleeping, difficulty thinking, and mood swings. This made it almost impossible for Joni to fulfill her work obligations. At first she kept pushing through, trying to tolerate the medicine, but since her quality of life was so diminished, she finally decided to live with the risk and was at peace with her decision.

Sometimes it is not just the cost-benefit analysis of one decision, sometimes you have to compare the outcome statistics of two choices. What would you do if you knew that a lumpectomy has a chance of cure in 90 percent of women, but a mastectomy has a chance of 95 percent? You will have to take other aspects into consideration. Can you live with the outcome when you choose a lumpectomy and happen to be the 1/10 unlucky women who will have a recurrence? Will you kick yourself that you should've chosen the mastectomy, even though you couldn't know at the time of the choice that you would be on the unlucky side of the draw? Or are you deciding based on fear and choose the safer option of mastectomy but didn't realize until after the fact that you're not happy with the cosmetic outcome? These are all incredibly difficult decision you have to make without ever knowing the outcome but having to live with whatever choice you make.

DEALING WITH STATISTICS

Mortality-Survival Statistics

You have probably had more than your fair share of statistics lessons, but I am afraid there is another important statistics-related topic we must discuss. Patients are usually given an XX-year survival rate, often five. What this statistic tells us is the number of people in a particular situation who will be alive after five years. The big problem with the number, as we saw earlier when discussing statistics, is that this tells us nothing about how you as an individual will fare.

Statistics are never about an individual; they're a look at whole groups. If I tell you that your five-year survival rate is 90 percent, most people will be happy, but that has to do with how humans hear. Remember our discussion of confirmation bias at the beginning of the book? We tend to listen for information that will confirm our existing beliefs. Most people hearing this stat will conclude that they will be alive in five years. Unfortunately this is not fact.

Jim dealt with the opposite problem. He had a rare form of lung cancer. After his diagnosis and treatment, the doctor told him that he had a 15 percent chance of being alive in two years. That was in fact a low probability. Only fifteen out of 100 people in Jim's situation would be alive in two years, and eighty-five out of 100 would be dead. Jim unfortunately interpreted that information to mean that he was going to be dead in two years. He only heard how low his chances were and concluded that he was going to be in the group of people who would be dead.

He could not imagine that he was the one who was going to be alive and he started to live accordingly. Believing he was going to be dead soon, he pretty much stopped living and waited for death to arrive.

This was over ten years ago, and Jim is still here. He was obviously wrong in his assumption/expectation, but the thought "I will be dead in two years" was so traumatic for Jim and kept him so distressed and sleepless that it took him a long time to recover emotionally. This is a good place to remind you of Bessel Van der Kolk's notion that the body keeps the score. Jim had been traumatized not by the statistical probability itself but by his misinterpretation of it. Not only did his body keep the score, feeling uncomfortable, but his mind also held onto the idea that he was going to be dead soon.

It took Jim a long time to believe that he would be the one to beat his lousy odds. When listening to your own numbers, always keep in mind that you do not know—in fact there is no way to know!—whether a particular outcome will be true for you.

Whatever the probabilities are or your situation, you need to remember that you simply don't know whether they will apply to you as an individual. And there is no way of knowing. This is very hard to get comfortable with. Here's the link again to a YouTube video that you can watch to help you get your head around this issue. (https://www.youtube.com/watch?v=PhX13NgDgxc&t=194s)

Disease-Free Statistics

Patients are also given probabilities of their chance of being cancer free after a certain number of years (again usually five). Again these statistics tell you nothing about what will happen to you!

If I tell you that you have a 90 percent chance of being cancer free in five years, you would probably be very happy. With our yearning for confirmation bias, most people hearing this number would conclude that they will be disease free in five years.

This was true for Elizabeth. Her numbers were even better. She was told that 99 percent of people in her situation will be cancer free after five years. Elizabeth interpreted that as a cure. She dutifully waited to have children for five years to make sure she was part of the cancer-free group. She resumed life, started a family, and settled into feeling cured. Ten years after her original diagnosis, however, disaster struck. Elizabeth was not just diagnosed with cancer again but with a metastasis of her original cancer.

This is the horror scenario that no one wants to even think about. Elizabeth was among the unlucky 1 percent who got sick again. She regretted deeply not having started a family right after her treatment was done. Fortunately for Elizabeth, the story has a happy ending. Despite her recurrence in another part of her body, her illness turned out to manageable. She is doing well, and both her children are in college.

But the story illustrates the human desire to create certainty. In Jim's example, he imagined certain death; in Elizabeth's example, she imagined a cure. And as you know already, both were wrong.

But where does that leave *you*? I present these unusual examples as an appeal to you to learn and practice living with uncertainty. To learn to envision both sides of the coin: *I am going to live now as if I am going to live a long life, but at the same time, I am going to live now as if I am not going to be alive a long time.*

This is where the one, five, ten, twenty-five-year exercise comes into play. Create a table like the one below and list all the activities you can't decide whether to do because you do not know how long you are going to live. Then speculate whether you would do the activity based on the projected lifespan. This is how it looks:

1-, 5-, 10-, 25-year Exercise Sample Table 7a

	If I am alive in …… I will/won't…..			
Activity	**1 year**	**5 year**	**10 year**	**25 year**
Go shopping today				
Fix the sink				
Make love to my partner today				
Replace windows in my house				
Look for a new job				
Move to a different apartment				
Cash in my 401k				

To illustrate the point, I picked activities of daily living, but it is important that you pick whatever is relevant for your own life. Below a blank of Table 7 for you to work on:

1-, 5-, 10-, 25-year Exercise Sample Blank Table 7b

	If I am alive in ...... I will/won't.....			
Activity	**1 year**	**5 year**	**10 year**	**25 year**

The results are usually quite illuminating. There are certain things you will do no matter how long your life span and others for which your projected lifespan might make a difference. Once you have identified the things on your list that might make a difference, you can strategically compromise both desires. And now you don't have to pay attention to the ones you determine don't matter anymore.

SLEEP DISTURBANCE

Not sleeping messes with pretty much everybody. Problems with falling asleep or daytime sleepiness affect thirty-five to 40 percent of U. S. adults, even without having cancer (Hossain & Shapiro, 2002). When you get sick, your chances of sleep disturbance go up. A study designed to explore whether medication decreases sleep problems in women with breast cancer who underwent chemotherapy reported that 88 percent of participants reported difficulty sleeping. That's pretty much everybody. The medicine did help, but 79 percent still reported trouble with sleeping, even on the medicine (Palesh et al., 2012). That is four out of five patients, even with medicine on board. That is way too many!

Sleep is a fickle creature, and sleeplessness serves as a sensitive indicator that something is amiss with your health. Distress frequently equals difficulty sleeping. Autonomic nervous system activation, either from positive excitement or unpleasant distress, keeps people awake. When you constantly need to be vigilant to run away from the lion, aka the cancer that is about to eat you, you don't sleep. We have touched on sleep several times in this book already because of its fundamental contribution to health.

Daniel Levitin, whose book *The Organized Mind* I mentioned in **Chapter 4** on **Thinking**, reports on how active our brain is at night while we sleep and how important sleep is to our capacity to cognitively process enormous amounts of information in order to help form and protect memories. If I had only one option to treat and could fulfill it with a genie wish, I would enable everybody to sleep better. Remember how in **Chapter 4 and 5** I hammered on the point that distress messes with your thinking and your emotions? Lack of sleep or poor sleep do pretty much the same thing (Walker, 2009).

Because this book is already long and the subject is so complex, I can only give you snippets of the importance of sleep. If you want to go deeper, I recommend reading *Why We Sleep*, also by Matthew Walker. It may be scary to read how affected our health is by lack of sleep, but rather than be afraid, take it as an inspiration to take the best possible care of sleep as you can.

My expertise is in helping people be as healthy as possible with as little medication as possible. Patients specifically seek me out for this skill, and I usually stay within the confines of the request. The one exception I make, however, regards sleep. I will occasionally push sleep medicine at people who do not want it (and of course I back off if they reject it). My patients know I mean business when I tilt my head, put on a stern look, and lean in: "Johnny, I know you want to accomplish this without medication, but if you don't sleep, it is not going to be the cancer that will kill you, it will be the lack of sleep. If you don't sleep, you cannot function. When we can't function, we make poor choices."

"Mary, you realize that not sleeping makes you a worse driver than driving drunk. You are about to make a decision to live without a body part that is fundamental to your identity. Would you want to make such a decision while dangerously drunk (Dement, 1997)?"

This might sound radical and pushy, but I've seen too often that people totally underestimate the importance of sleep and don't realize the price they pay. It's not that I want to push, but this is one of those lesser of two evils questions you have to answer for yourself, not unlike some of the other suboptimal medical decision choices we discussed earlier. Sometimes there is no good choice, just a less bad one. So ask yourself if it's less bad to forego medication and not to sleep at all or to sleep a little bit with some.

To make sound choices about your treatment, you need to be at your best cognitively. After the initial shock of diagnosis, patients will often look for optimal treatment and are faced with a variety of important choices regarding treatment, as well as finding a suitable treating team. In this phase, many patients are in cognitive overdrive, trying to optimize choices that they are often not equipped to judge medically. This leads to thought intrusion and thought flooding and often their companion, difficulty sleeping.

Here I want to remind you that, like emotions, thoughts are state dependent. As we discussed in **Chapter 4** on **Thinking**, thoughts can take on a life of their own. At night thoughts tend to get distorted even more than during the day. We can experience a problem as suffocating and impossible to solve when we think about it in the fearful dark of the night, but the same exact issue seems manageable after a cup of tea in the morning in the presence of loving family or your dog. Adequate restful sleep will result in better thinking and better decision-making ability. The motive to think is problem solving, but if it happens at 2 A.M., the price you pay the next day is too high, particularly if the thinking at night does not produce a solution.

It is easy to find yourself in a vicious cycle of not sleeping at night because of thought hyperactivity, leading to exhaustion with limited problem-solving ability, which feeds into feeling overwhelmed and distressed, resulting in even worse problems sleeping. This is the reason I encourage patients to always assess whether their thinking constitutes problem-solving. If it only represents head spinning, it is not worth it. You are much better off picking a parasympathetic exercise and postponing thinking to a more functional time.

Reducing sympathetic and increasing parasympathetic tone is at the core of successfully sleeping. We learned earlier that the parasympathetic nervous system is responsible for "rest and digest." Sleep functions to restore brain chemicals the body needs to operate at its best the next day. And this is why I sometimes push medication. Whatever it takes, you need to sleep. Even at the price that some of these medications will influence your sleep quality. Here we are again at a cost-benefit analysis regarding decision-making, much like the one I introduced a couple of sections ago. Better did you get some mediocre sleep than no sleep at all.

For patients who are adamant about not wanting to take medication, there are many alternatives in the complementary and integrative medicine toolbox. Yoga, acupuncture, massage, biofeedback, and meditation are among many options that seem to have beneficial effects (Sarris & Byrne, 2011).

CONSIDER THE STAGE AND TYPE OF CANCER YOU HAVE

When considering your options and decisions, the single most important advice I can give you is not to mix apples and oranges. If you meet someone who also has cancer, there is a reasonable chance that your illnesses have little overlap the same way, that there is nothing much similar about being a line cook and a housekeeper, even though you might both work in the hospitality industry. Cancer is the umbrella term for a huge variation of illnesses with very different symptoms, causes, treatments, and outcomes. Using the word "cancer" does not do justice to this wide variety of conditions. It's like saying that you own a vehicle without differentiating between a tricycle or a Lamborghini. As we discussed earlier in **Chapter 5** on **Emotions** in the section **Emotions Under Duress 2.0**, the word "cancer" itself evokes much emotion, even when you meet someone with a totally different medical situation, your emotional brain might still jump off the deep end. When that happens, try to not reason with the intensity but engage in any of the exercises in this book that help you center yourself. Take a deep breath and say, "What happens to person X is different from what happens to me, even though the feelings might be similarly scary," followed by a deep breath and the sentence "Emotions can be very intense when they're fueled by fear." Just acknowledging that you are different from person X will help the body mellow. Your options and decisions are unique to your diagnosis. Try not to let other people's experiences with other types of cancer intrude.

As we have talked about the many challenges of the diagnostic phase before the actual treatment, let's move on to the next part of the process.

CHAPTER 12.

Managing Treatment

I am often surprised and amazed at how emotionally stable people are during treatment. With life as they know it on hold, they have a singular focus on getting through treatment. They're in action mode. During treatment you're also probably getting the most help and support. There is an end in sight and a defined timeframe. Even though you will probably have to deal with the numerous side effects and possible complications of treatment, feeling poorly is no surprise.

But sometimes people bite off more than they can chew with respect to working while being sick. Having an illness is a full-time job. To go from one job to two jobs and not feel physically well is more than most people can handle. Peter did not tolerate his chemotherapy, and as a result, could not work. This affected his mood as his ability to work was very important to him. His identity had been rooted in his profession and being the provider for his family. The physical symptoms, including neuropathy and hiccups, also prevented him from sleeping. As a result, he could also not function at home, and this previously competent and engaging man fell apart emotionally. It's really important to get professional guidance in these situations, it can be so helpful. What Peter needed was to understand clearly that cancer had temporarily become his job, and his treatment-related symptoms did not allow for a second one. That allowed him to focus on getting better, not feeling like a loser, and to resume where he had left off after he had healed.

If you find yourself in this situation, I urge you to seek out palliative care. Despite increasing education and information, patients and caregivers still think of palliative care as "hospice." When I suggest it, people will often ask, "Am I dying?" While it is true that palliative care has a great role to play for the dying, that is not its sole function. The goal of palliative care is to provide relief from the symptoms and stress of a serious illness in order to improve quality of life for both the patient and the family.

One study I often refer to shows people that something good can come of early palliative care (Temel et al., 2010). Even though the study did address palliative care in the context of metastatic illness, the beautiful finding was that the people who received palliative care early on lived longer. I want you to take this to heart, even if you don't have metastatic illness, because taking care of your pain, sleep, nausea, bowel movements, and emotions will help getting you through your cancer treatment with greater ease. If you choose not to seek palliative care, please be sure to address the side effects of your treatment as much as possible with your surgeon, oncologist, or radiation oncologist.

Receiving treatment for cancer is not a cakewalk. and finding ways to be as comfortable as possible during treatment will help you get through it.

Fatigue, pain, cognitive problems, lack of energy, sleeplessness—these are all part of being in treatment, and I will describe these issues in more detail in **Chapter 13** on **Survivorship: Life after Treatment**. The symptoms themselves will be very similar during and after treatment, but your expectations will differ widely. As we discussed earlier in this chapter, symptoms make treatment hard, but knowing it only lasts for a finite time usually helps people buckle down and endure whatever comes their way. After treatment, however, patients often have less tolerance for those same symptoms because they don't expect them and they get in the way of resuming life. Living with symptoms with an unknown expiration date is not exactly a morale booster. But more on this in the next chapter.

But if you are currently going through treatment and are struggling with the many side effects, please try to apply the techniques I will describe in **Chapter 13**. The treatment to alleviate them are the same.

I do want to mention here though, something about the common response to the specific circumstances of radiation treatment. These days radiation is so precise that they literally have to tie you down, so you won't move while you're being treated. While this is for the patient's own benefit, it can be very hard to feel trapped like that, as if there is no escape. Cancer itself is already an out-of-control experience; being restrained on top of it can evoke quite a bit of distress.

Depending on your philosophy, you can either treat yourself to benzodiazepines—in collaboration with your doctor of course—or use techniques such as guided imagery or self-hypnosis to alleviate the distress. You might've experienced a similar unpleasantness when getting an MRI, where you also could not move, but with radiation, the sensation is more pronounced since you are literally tied down (depending on the body part that gets radiated).

Again my point is you don't need to tough it out. Medication and other interventions can really help reduce your distress. And I think we can all agree that one thing you don't need is to upset you more.

You might wonder why this chapter on managing treatment is so short since your medical treatment is the main point, but from an emotional perspective, other parts and phases of your illness and treatment will weigh more heavily on you.

CHAPTER 13.

Survivorship: Life after Treatment

It's time we look at survivorship. That term is usually used to describe the time from diagnosis forward, but that includes everyone experiencing cancer, from diagnosis to cure to death. I will use it more narrowly to talk about those who are at the end of treatment and have been declared in remission or "cancer free." People in this group will have a different emotional experience from someone with metastatic cancer, whose experience I will address in **Chapter 16** on **Living with Illness**.

I don't love the term "survivorship," but it has established itself, so I will use it, albeit in this modified version. The reservation I have is that we perceive cancer differently from heart disease or diabetes. We don't talk about a heart attack survivor or a diabetes survivor, even though both illnesses disable and kill. And many people survive them, just as they do cancer. It's a misleading distinction.

The potentially heart-wrenching journey of survivorship is eloquently described in a 2015 article in the *New York Times* by Suleika Jaouad, in which she describes the physical and emotional aftermath of cancer and the process of adapting. Her articulate piece also describes poignantly how follow-up care for cancer-related problems is often not accessible. People are closely monitored and tended to during treatment, but after treatment, it's a different story.

Fortunately more and more cancer centers recognize that people who are cured will continue to need physical and emotional support after the end of treatment. If you have access to such a survivorship program, take advantage of it, even only to help you not forget that you need basic health care and prevention for the rest of your body, which gets easily forgotten in the tunnel vision focus on cancer after cancer.

A lot of the struggles in this phase have to do with your expectations. As I was digging through the literature to check my belief that having low expectations comes with less disappointment if the expectations are not fulfilled, and higher expectations lead to higher disappointment if the expectations are not fulfilled, I had to admit that the relationship between expectations and satisfaction does not seem to be as direct and simple as I wanted it to be. As usual you have to figure out how *you* experience this post-treatment phase. For some people, cancer grants inspiration to find a different sense of meaning and purpose, but for others, the task of rebuilding their life is deeply unsettling. If I had to sum up survivorship in one sentence: "The old feels wrong, and the new has not arrived yet." While patients at the time of diagnosis yank up the coping strategies they are best at, even if they don't apply to the situation at hand, this approach rarely works during survivorship. The following sections present the major issues I have observed clinically and offers some suggestions to help with the reorientation.

RESUMING LIFE

Right after treatment, many people feel considerable relief. They expect immediate improvement and being able to resume their previous life. As you reintegrate, however, you will discover that healing takes time, and the post treatment period comes with considerable adjustments. People experience a slew of symptoms. Pain and aches are immediately misinterpreted as cancer related. Sleep feels elusive. Family and friends seem strangely altered. Superiors at work appear unsupportive.

The shock of the experience, treatment-related changes, and a different outlook on life make many patients question their judgment. To be able to put your experience in perspective requires distance, healing, and time. Over time cancer survivors will usually feel more optimistic and joyful. If you struggle in this phase, please seek help from providers with experience in such matters. An integrative oncologist or psycho-oncologist might be able to help depending on your symptom profile. If you want to work through it yourself, know that doing so will require you to balance maintaining hope for improvement and taking actions that will facilitate that improvement while also learning to adapt to the reality that not everything will be the way it was before.

Orient yourself toward actions that will facilitate improvement and overall well-being while at the same time developing a capacity to tolerate change and adjustment. You might want to revisit the concept of emotional agility. I like Susan David's approach of orienting yourself towards value-based actions. I agree with her that it is a mood and tolerance booster.

CAUSALITY IN SURVIVORSHIP

Just as you probably grappled with causality in the diagnostic phase, it comes up again in survivorship. You may wish to be flawless in your behavior and want to absolutely do everything right to make sure the cancer *never* comes back. This sometimes leads people to extreme diets and lifestyle changes. Personally I believe moderation in behavior and promoting emotional well-being are the key points, but there is extensive literature on how to live after cancer.

The book *Anti-Cancer* by David Servan-Schreiber holds many practical options for patients who want to be proactive in this area. Whatever you decide, if it comes from a center of emotional well-being, it cannot be wrong as a peaceful feeling allows for a parasympathetic tone, which itself is conducive to health and healthier choices. In other words, please don't trap yourself into thinking one false move and you'll be dealing with cancer again. Fortunately, and unfortunately, there is no direct line between our behavior choices and health outcomes. And please do seek out resources to help you live well after cancer.

COGNITIVE FUNCTION

Changes in cognitive function and what to do about them are a huge topic of discussion in cancer care. While cognitive symptoms are reported at the time of diagnosis and during treatment (Wefel et al., 2015), I decided to place the discussion here because changes in your thinking can become life-limiting after cancer, and more so if they're unexpected. During treatment people tend to be more tolerant of being cognitively slow and reduced, but after the completion of treatment, you want to reintegrate into life and resume normalcy, and you expect functionality.

As we discussed in **Chapter 4** on **Thinking**, cognition is more than just thinking. Cognition includes perceiving, processing, and retaining information. Cognition helps with focus and attention. All these functions can be disturbed in the cancer experience. People complain about difficulty focusing, difficulty concentrating, and difficulty remembering. Commonly this is called "chemobrain," but you'll remember from earlier discussions that it's not just the chemotherapy that messes with your brain but the distress you experience while you deal with cancer.

We already met Diana, a lawyer, in **Chapter 6** on **Body**. She had experienced herself as a "brain on a stick" prior to getting sick. She took for granted her ability to juggle numerous legal projects concurrently. After treatment the one and only organ she had cared about all her life, her brain, let her down. Linda reported concern with memory also. She repeated questions without realizing it until she was reminded that her question had already previously been answered. She accidentally recycled her credit card, absentmindedly carrying it to the recycling bin and then desperately searched for it in her house, not remembering what she'd done. Linda had prided herself on productivity and efficiency; not being able to execute on her thoughts and expectations was very stressful. Linda expressed concern that she might be developing Alzheimer's at the age of forty-one!

Even though patients have long reported cognitive problems, chemobrain was not a recognized entity in medicine for a very long time. Physicians would only accept that cancer in the brain itself could cause difficulty but not cancer outside the brain. They reasoned that chemotherapy could not possibly affect cognition, since many of these medications cannot enter the brain from the bloodstream. "It is just in your head" was a common attitude that caused patients unnecessary emotional suffering.

As we learned earlier, "The science of today is often the error of tomorrow." This is definitely true in the area of cognitive dysfunction in cancer patients. The saying would in fact more accurately be, "The science of yesterday turned out to be the error of yesterday."

Fortunately research has helped us make much progress in our understanding of this issue. Numbers vary, but estimates are that up to 60 percent of patients report changes in cognition after cancer (Janelsins et al., 2014). Most of the data stem from patients who underwent chemotherapy, but there are reports that patients can experience cognitive dysfunction without chemotherapy, raising speculations that cancer itself might be the culprit.

Animal studies suggest that the hippocampus, the part of the brain responsible for helping memory, is affected in cancer. This might be related to the fact that stress and inflammation decrease the body's ability to build the nerve cells necessary for thinking. A thorough explanation of the science is beyond the scope of this book, but clinicians and deep-diving patients can explore a summary article for evidence and information (Wefel et al., 2015).

If you want to be proactive, you can get neurocognitive testing and neurocognitive rehabilitation. Unfortunately the test may not show much, as there seems to be a discrepancy between what you experience and what shows up on the test (Lange et al., 2019), but don't let that deter you from taking your symptoms seriously. The authors of the article cited just above point to this: "cognitive functioning is affected in day-to-day life, but compensatory mechanisms maintain performance in the structured, distraction-free environment of neuropsychological testing" as a possible explanation for the discrepancy. They also point out that other factors, such as depression or insomnia, can affect testing and performance.

You might find the book *Improving Cognitive Function After Cancer* by Shelli Kesler helpful. The take-home message for the reader is clear: "It is definitely in your head but not the way you were made to believe." Difficulty with cognition related to cancer and its treatment is real and not a product of your imagination. If someone tells you that your symptoms are psychosomatic, remember that they are really somatic. They might affect your psyche and your emotions, but they're definitely not imagined. They are due to a process happening in your body (i.e. somatic) that has eluded scientific explanations so far. Which does not mean they are not real or not present. Remember that what we observe is not nature itself but nature exposed to our methods of questioning, as I quoted Werner Heisenberg earlier. What is going on in your brain and what you perceive is real, but the tests to assess your symptoms might not always be sensitive enough to pick it up.

If you want to explore neurocognitive rehabilitation, those programs are successful (Bray et al., 2017), the same way physical therapy helps heal a twisted ankle. If it is available to you, it is worth pursuing to find out how it works for you.

FATIGUE

Like cognitive issues, fatigue is very common in cancer patients. Depending on which literature and surveys you look at, somewhere between 50 percent and 90 percent of patients experience fatigue during and after cancer treatment (Ebede et al., 2017). No matter which data you consider, that's a lot of people. The tiredness, inactivity, weakness, and exhaustion are pronounced and out of proportion to the activities you're engaging in. You feel excessively fatigued despite doing very little, and the fact that this fatigue interferes with daily functioning adds its own stress. Bear in mind we're not talking about lofty goals of climbing Kilimanjaro but climbing out of bed to make your children breakfast.

There is a lot of overlap between cognitive dysfunction and fatigue, and they also feed on each other. If the fatigue mostly affects brain function, with reduced concentration and capacity for paying attention or retaining new information, these are symptoms identical to cognitive ones. Linda, whom we discussed in the discussion of cognitive dysfunction, worried that she had Alzheimer's. Patients who feel distracted or can't retain information sometimes decide that they have attention deficit disorder. They have neither Alzheimer's nor attention deficit disorder, but with symptoms so debilitating, it's easy to understand why people would come to these conclusions.

Brian, a high functioning executive in the computer business, is someone who experienced both cognitive difficulty and debilitating fatigue in an unrelenting way. He described being at about 30 percent of prior mental acuity. He used to love solving his work-related computer riddles way into the night, feeling energized by the challenge. Now, however, he was so tired throughout the day that he often needed to take naps at work. Fortunately his employer was very supportive. His manager placed a couch in Brian's office to help him stay functional. Despite all the support, Brian needed to retire after two years of agony.

He had been declared cured of cancer by his oncologist, but he felt far from healthy. In fact he reported that if he could choose a do-over, he would prefer to forgo treatment and die from cancer. While from a medical perspective, he had won the lottery, a cure, he did not consider the benefit worth the cost. Please understand that the radicalness of his view was a reflection of the degree of his suffering, not a desire to die.

Brian had been physically and mentally thriving before his cancer diagnosis. For some people, the complicated blend of fatigue and difficulty thinking that accompanies their cancer makes them realize that they had similar symptoms before as elements of burnout. It can be difficult to distinguish between post-cancer blues and pre-cancer burnout catching up with someone. Feeling physically tired and emotionally exhausted and not performing up to standard are common in both. People will often start to question their abilities and lose perspective about the future. Paired with pain and difficulty sleeping, this blend can lead to depression.

Something that complicated Brian's experience was that his decline was real and debilitating, but because his pre-cancer performance was off the charts, he was terribly frustrated when neurocognitive testing did not reveal any pathology. In his case, it was all relative. Compared to the performance of the rest of the population, he was still a star, but he felt inadequate because he knew what he'd been capable of and no longer was.

Unfortunately cognitive decline is rarely documented because very few patients receive testing before treatment. Remember the section on normal distribution?

If you want to practice more of the exercises you learned in **Chapter 9**, Figure 24 shows Brian's conundrum. To Brian's surprise, he performed above average compared to the whole population on neurocognitive testing, but *his* actual decline could not be documented since he had no pretreatment baseline.

Figure 24

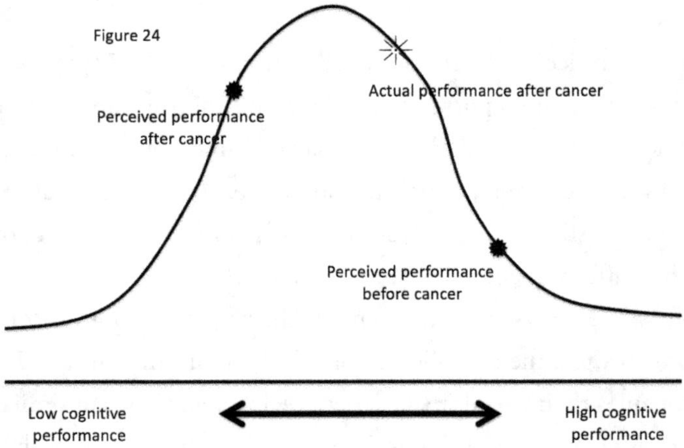

It wasn't his actual performance that was the problem but the difference of his perception, which resulted in the long distance on the bell curve. By his employer's standards, he was performing just fine. In fact they were so eager to have him that they didn't mind the daily nap in the office. But this did not console Brian or help make him feel adequate. If you apply this exercise to yourself, remember that the distance on the bell curve will be the determining factor for the distress you will feel.

People in highly cognitive professions often share Brian's fate. To the outside world, they look and perform fine, but they know that they have declined, and the difference feels too great. Being able to take naps on the couch at work did help but ultimately did not solve Brian's problem. In addition to frustration about his lower performance, his sense of self, which was so deeply rooted in success and performance, took a hit and contributed to the fatigue and difficulty thinking. To restore energy and maintain it takes patience, and after enduring arduous treatment, the disappointment of a prolonged recovery can be devastating.

SLEEP DISTURBANCE

I mention sleep disturbance again here as I did in **Chapter 11** on **Dealing With Diagnosis**. Difficulty with sleep is an ongoing problem for many, not just at the time of diagnosis but during treatment and after treatment. Adding difficulty sleeping into the mix of cognitive difficulty and fatigue can throw people over the edge.

Joni's employer was not as understanding as Brian's. She lost her job as a lawyer and got to the brink of suicide. An endless, vicious cycle of fatigue feeding on difficulty concentrating, feeding on distress, feeding on not sleeping, feeding on waking up exhausted in the morning, feeding on not being able to perform keeps a relentless cycle going. The issues are very similar to what I described in **Chapter 11** in the section on **Sleep Disturbance**, and I recommend that you reread it. Once again reducing sympathetic and increase parasympathetic tone is at the core of successfully sleeping.

The big difference between sleeplessness from the time of diagnosis and treatment and sleeplessness after cancer is that after cancer, people wonder if it will ever get better. People in survivorship sometimes lose hope and cannot imagine an end to sleeplessness and low-quality sleep. Survivorship, unlike treatment itself, has no defined end, and as we have learned, we humans are not good with uncertainty. So in addition to practicing the recommendations in **Chapter 11** to help you sleep, I also want you to practice what I prescribed for dealing with uncertainty. Please reread **Chapter 8** to be reminded of practices you can do every day to minimize the distress of uncertainty, so you can focus on your parasympathetic activities to improve your sleep. *Control* and *Caregiving* were needs you looked at in previous algorithm exercises. Revisit Figure 20, but this time with the need for *certainty*.

SYMPATHETIC HYPERAROUSAL

I hope by now you have burned the expression sympathetic hyperarousal into your brain as a factor that contributes a lot to the havoc of what happens not just during cancer but post-cancer. We have seen how distress is an exacerbating factor of cognitive difficulty, sleep disturbance, and fatigue. Linda's symptoms of misplacing things, forgetting, and spacing out were not based on early dementia but were likely cognitive changes related to cancer and treatment. She described how she would constantly *think* about doing things but not actually do them, and despite the lack of action, still felt rushed and hurried. What Linda described post-cancer was sympathetic hyperarousal based on stressful thought. She cognitively overstimulated herself and had no mental reserve to perceive and process. Once Linda was aware of the association, she started to do specific exercises aimed at reducing stress, as well as exercises to strengthen her cognitive function.

If you feel that these might help you, you can go back to **Chapter 4** on **Thinking** and reread the parts about how sympathetic activation messes with your brain, then revisit the exercises, which might help you to not feel so much at the mercy of your body going in terror mode.

PAIN

Hundreds, if not thousands, of books have been written about how to best assess and treat pain. In this section, I am only focusing on what might trip you up emotionally when you feel pain during survivorship and make suggestions so your distress about pain doesn't make things worse.

The price of treatment can often be pain. The causes vary. In a study of forty women who were between six months and five years post-breast cancer diagnosis, 68 percent reported that pain was interfering with their life, and 63 percent had a pain intensity higher than what someone who did not go through cancer would experience (Schreier et al., 2019). The data is scary but also points at the importance of tending to pain in the survivorship phase.

Like fatigue, insomnia, and other symptoms mentioned in **Chapter 12** on **Managing Treatment**, cancer patients buckle down through anything while going through treatment, but once the active phase of treatment is over, the reality of not returning to normalcy and acceptable health hits hard. Pain has a similar impact.

This unfortunately also coincides with less frequent contact with health care providers. Dealing with symptoms, not always knowing how to best treat them, and not being embedded in an active treatment team with almost daily access can be sobering and overwhelming. A further challenge is prescription medication. While pain medication is generously prescribed during treatment, prescriptions are handled more restrictively in the survivorship phase because some of them carry a risk of dependency. Another complication is people's tendency to misinterpreted pain as a recurrence of cancer. The key word here to remember is interoception, the ability (but unfortunately sometimes also inability) of the brain to perceive, process, and integrate the senses from within the body. What can you do when the brain concludes that pain signaled to the brain is cancer, even when it isn't?

First of all, take advantage of the arsenal of treatments available to you to treat your pain as best as possible, including pain management clinics, acupuncture, hypnosis, and physical therapy to name a few. But most importantly, from the perspective of cancer distress, pain is the ultimate teacher of living with uncertainty. While you pursue treatment, you also must get comfortable with adaptation to pain. To juggle and reconcile these opposite ideas in the same universe is hard. I sound like a broken record, but practicing exercises from previous chapters can help. **Chapter 8** and **9** hold practices you can do every day to minimize the distress of uncertainty, so you can focus on your parasympathetic activities to improve pain. Table 2 in **Chapter 6** lists suggestions that might suit you. Some of them are proven to be effective treatments for pain, even without the associated distress of pain (Nahin et al., 2016). Pretty much any exercise in this book will do.

It probably isn't a consolation but taking little steps and reminding yourself of the parallel process of adaptation to pain and pursuing steps to treat it does help. And it won't take 10,000 hours to accomplish. Chip away at it one minute at a time. One minute here and there while you carry the awareness for what seems mutually exclusive needs. A brief meditation on the sentence: "I don't know what the future brings, but I wonder what (feasible) action I could take right now that has a chance at easing my pain in this minute or at least focus on something that isn't as preoccupying." Or: "I wonder if I can allow myself to tend to my pain for just one minute by taking a deep breath, re-orienting my thoughts towards the present rather than the fear of the future and letting my gaze stare at the landscape of wherever I am right now." And of course, as is second nature by now, these sentences are accompanied by you taking slow deep breaths.

FEAR OF RECURRENCE

Revisiting the grooved thinking mentioned in the introduction, let's acknowledge again how difficult it is to change thinking. When discussing that aspect with patients, I often meet with resistance. Some patients experience their thinking as a warning system. Pain often triggers the chain of thoughts that gets your nervous system going in this department.

When Daisy tells me that "thinking that a physical symptom could represent cancer, even when everybody tells me it is not, I am on the appropriate alert to catch the cancer when it comes back," I understand her purpose. When John tells me that before he goes to sleep, "rattling down a list of all the things that happened in a day and thinking about all the things that can happen the next day, I will be better prepared to handle the following day and finally feel some peace," I understand his intentions as well. Both of them are expressing a desire for preparedness and peace and staying alert and thinking methodically are attempts at achieving them.

I usually cannot convince people to abstain from that thinking unless I can convince them that they pay too high a price for their approach. In the cost-benefit analysis, there is definitely a benefit, but the cost is quite high. When looking at the diagram of cognition, body, and emotion, we understand easily that these thoughts fulfill needs, but they come at the price of stress. Daisy will activate her body with her thinking because her body is now more on alert for physical symptoms, and John probably will have a hard time going to sleep with his bedtime routine. But when Daisy and John realize that they can accomplish some peace and preparedness without making their bodies stressed in the process, the seed of collaboration and success is sown.

If Daisy can tell herself that she thinks about her symptoms to fulfill her need for safety and preparedness, she might more easily be able to acknowledge that at the same time that thought is making her anxious and stressed. Her desire to find peace is understandable, but she has not realized that her attempt comes at a price, which is stress on her body and her mind. Similarly John is trying to organize his mind in preparation for the next day and does not realize that the same activity that is supposed to bring him peace is bringing the sleepless night and exhaustion the next day.

If we understand the connection, we have room for alternatives and negotiations. We can brainstorm about activities that bring peace and safety *without* the body paying a price, and in the best-case scenario, we can even find a way to calm the body and go to sleep *while* finding peace and safety or whatever it is we need at that time. This exercise takes practice, but it is worthwhile as it caters to at least the optimizers among us.

TRIGGERS DURING THE SURVIVORSHIP PHASE

Other People's Stories

A patient tells me she had been doing well with respect to her own health, but then when a co-worker diagnosed with cancer seven years ago recently died, she got concerned about her own situation. She says that not knowing about her prognosis makes her focused on how to live life in a meaningful way. Anything in that realm can be a trigger: hearing about another person's illness, witnessing a friend's or even stranger's illness, dealing with the illness of a loved one. There isn't really an association between the significance of the person and your response. Your brain hears the word "cancer," and it'll explode.

We had talked about the brain's tendency to misinterpret when it is distressed. It is indeed very difficult to not confuse someone else's cancer with your own. Try to be generous with the frailty of your brain when it comes to what constitutes a stress response to the word cancer. Remind yourself of Bessel Van der Kolk's analogy to a smoke detector I mentioned in **Chapter 5** in the section on **Emotion-Associated Actions**. We want the smoke detector to alert us to a potential fire, but it will also go off with a smoky oven. When you are distressed, you tend to misinterpret the cause of the alarm and have a diminished ability to differentiate between different levels of danger. You feel an urge to call 911, even if you are dealing with burnt cookies and not a burning house. The brain translates "Mary has cancer" to "my cancer will come back, or my cancer will kill me." Take a deep breath so the brain can regroup and separate Mary's story from yours.

Other People's Responses

We have already looked at how difficult it can be to deal with other people's responses to your diagnosis. This is no different after you are done with treatment. Friends and coworkers will assume that your life will go back to normal. They share your wish for it to be so. But with high expectations can come big disappointment. This often leads to conflict.

Celeste had always been outgoing. The center of every party. Friends would come to her house after work, socialize, watch TV, and help each other. Celeste was looking forward to resuming a normal life. However, it was not meant to be. Ongoing treatment left her with hot flashes, difficulty sleeping, difficulty with memory and concentration. She felt always exhausted and wasn't in the mood to socialize. This took everybody by surprise, most of all Celeste. She felt guilty that she couldn't accommodate her friends who tried to push her to resume the precancer gatherings. Only with gradual acceptance of the changes and slow integration with some limited activities that felt appealing could Celeste resume some sense of normalcy. Sadly many of her old friends could not adjust with her, and old connections came to an end.

Surveillance

How to monitor one's health without living in constant fear is something that trips up many patients. How often do you want to check if anything cancer related might be happening inside? Patients often struggle with how often and how to undertake what's commonly called post cancer *surveillance*. While people are usually given guidelines to address the frequency with which to get a colonoscopy or mammogram, once cancer has visited you, the guidelines don't seem to appease your fear. I see people at both ends of the spectrum: patients who want frequent blood draws or to make their home in the lab to stay on top of things and others who don't want to look at all and rely on physical symptoms to remind them that something might be amiss in their body. But even patients who want frequent or regular surveillance go through a stressful time prior to the scheduled scan or venipuncture as it draws closer. Naturally your nervous system gets activated by the fear of what might await you, and it can be really challenging to stay levelheaded.

My advice as usual is to be as calm and clearheaded as possible as that improves well-being and decision-making. And I'm known for having my patients do mental multiplication tables while standing on one leg as they pretend to wait in the changing area. As you recall, you can crowd out your fearful thinking and the distress that is associated with it by focusing on something that gives the brain at least 120 bits per second of mental activity. If you need a refresher, revisit the section **The Brain, the Slowpoke** in **Chapter 4**.

Physical Symptoms

Physical symptoms, foremost pain, also have a very high probability of triggering your autonomic nervous system. How are you supposed to know whether your headache is due to tension or a recurrence of your brain tumor? How are you supposed to differentiate between an upset stomach and the recurrence of ovarian cancer? To find a mental space in which you are comfortable, determining when and how to evaluate is not always easy.

The common rule of waiting two weeks with a symptom to see if it will dissipate on its own is far easier said than done. People frequently have concerns related to the unpredictability and uncertainty of possible illness progression and (once again) will often respond to uncertainty with distress and lose their ability to evaluate their physical symptoms objectively. And if you are someone like Geoffrey—the unfortunate young man with tongue cancer—whose diagnosis took a long time, even if you get to survive your cancer, the fear of the delayed diagnosis sits deeply.

It can be really difficult to be objective in evaluating whether your physical symptoms are signs of serious illness. We're often not good judges of what to evaluate further. You might have perfect intellectual insight into this dynamic but still cannot manage to decrease stress around this experience. And you're probably tired of hearing it by now. If you improve your ability to induce a parasympathetic tone, the quality of your thoughts will improve with it, and that alone will help you make a risk-based assessment rather than a fear-based assessment.

CHAPTER 14.

Caregivers Unite

While a doctor is a caregiver in the general meaning of the word, the word in this book refers to those closest to the patient and involved in their care—a spouse, a relative, a close friend. While there are many lovely stories in which tangible and emotional support nicely matchup between caregiver and care receiver, there are as many that are illustrations for cause of pain and added distress. The vast majority of caregivers have the wonderful motivation of wanting to help, but that desire unfortunately is not enough to turn it into effective action of help. The desire to help does not automatically endow a person with the knowledge of how to successfully do it. The difficulty lies in part in the differences between the realities of the patient and of the world around the patient. And as is so often the case, when it gets dicey, it usually comes down to competing needs.

In **Chapter 9**, we looked at how "needs" covers a wide range of expression and differences, and when they clash between two parties, it gets tough. Nowhere is this more true than between caretakers and patients. Like doctors, family and friends often cannot truly relate to what it feels like to be a patient. This can lead to lack of understanding, well-meant but ineffective action, and sometimes even to pressuring a person to undergo interventions that will prolong their life, even when that would come at a horrendous price in terms of suffering and quality of life.

UNDERSTANDING

A caregiver's lack of understanding, as we've seen, can be very painful. In **Chapter 11** on **Dealing with Diagnosis**, we discussed that when people who are ill share not just the facts of what is happening to them but also how they feel about it, they will be met with a wide range of responses, many of them in the not-understanding-and-inappropriately-responding category. You might have to hear someone tell you that you don't feel the way you say you do. Even when they acknowledge that you do feel the way you say you do, they might tell you that what you are feeling is not such a big deal. And even when they acknowledge that what you're feeling is a big deal, they'll try to console you with offerings like "things will be better soon" (even when they won't). Most people find it very challenging to sit with someone else's simple expression of distress. They're uncomfortable with not knowing what to say or do. To make matters even trickier, people will often try to help in truly unhelpful ways.

This chapter is an appeal to caregivers to turn inward to evaluate their motivations and abilities and an appeal to patients to be emotionally generous with their caregivers and ultimately an appeal to both to communicate as openly as possible about these delicate matters. Unfortunately it is also an appeal to accept that the relationship might break down over differences in needs and abilities to give and receive.

THE HELPLESS HELPER

Most patients need help. Many people want to help. Which makes it all the more painful when caregiving turns into a contentious battle and endless source of disappointment. When I try to help bridge the chasm between their understandings of what constitutes help, I am pained by the added distress both parties experience. And all this is usually happening at a time when everybody needs an emotional break.

I had quoted one of the public eavesdropping clips in the *San Francisco Chronicle* earlier: "I'm not bossy. I'm just aggressively helpful," covers one end of the spectrum of the wrong help, with too much intensity, possibly even at the wrong time. Through the helper's eyes though, they are doing fine. This relativity in perception is something many cancer patients have to contend with. You are supposed to be grateful for what the helper can give, even when it is not what you need.

This topic is bound to hurt, puzzle, or anger the caregivers among you, so I am going to hide behind a paragraph from a book to illustrate. As you read the following, I ask that you try your hardest not to react but simply keep your mind open. The paragraph comes from a very moving book called *The Bright Hour*, written by Nina Riggs, who has since succumbed to cancer at a very young age. In one part, she is brainstorming with her friend who also has cancer about ideas for "morbid prefab cancer patient thank-you cards to real and imaginary people." This is what they came up with.

Thank you for the taco casserole. It worked even better than my stool softener.

Thoughts and prayers are great, but Ativan and pot are better.

Thank you for the flowers. I hope they die before I do.

All your phone messages about how not knowing exactly what's going on with me has stressed you out really help me put things in perspective.

Xanax is white, Zofran is blue, steroids make me feel like throttling you.

If you're the person trying to help, these words may hurt, but don't retreat. Your main job as a caregiver is to be in the service to the other person. This includes surrendering your own needs at times and being a student of what it means to be truly helpful. And that is, as many things, easier said than done.

Please don't hear this to mean that you're supposed to surrender all your needs all the time, or go so far beyond the call of duty that you exhaust yourself in care. This is not what I am (or Nina Riggs is) saying at all. What she's saying, in fact, is stay within the realm of your possibilities. Caretakers often confuse helping and serving with 24/7 availability. I often see caretakers go beyond their abilities and either break down or become resentful. To be realistic about what you can (and can't) do is more helpful to the patient than going beyond your abilities or giving something that's not wanted or needed. To give the wrong thing can be as painful or even worse to the patient as getting nothing.

That's what this imaginary thank-you note is really about. It is a sarcastic expression of what it feels like to get the wrong thing, the point being that your motive to help did not result in efficacious action that was perceived as helpful. It is important to differentiate between intent and action.

I have had heated discussions on this topic. I know people who think that intent should be given more value, and the action is not relevant. I strongly disagree. My disputants argue that you can throw out the tuna casserole or feed it to the dog if it does not please you. This, however, allows the giver not to take a decent measure of responsibility for their actions. If you're frugal, you will not throw out food, and as a recipient, you don't want to offend. Good intentions are not always enough.

Once again the devil is in the details. It's up to both of you to bridge the divide with openness, gentleness, tolerance, and gratitude. Imagine the bell curve. Even if you reside on opposite ends of the curve, you can at least communicate the issue peacefully and constructively. And when in doubt, the responsibility falls more heavily on the giver, especially if the receiver is very sick and needs to focus on their healing. As a patient, don't feel "selfish" and allow yourself to set boundaries. When Ronald K. Brown, a contemporary choreographer and dancer, suffered a stroke, his family suggested not to make an announcement on social media, telling him, "you don't want people coming out of the woodwork, wanting to come to the hospital or wanting to bring you food" (Kourlas, *New York Times*, March 6, 2022). They had the foresight to protect him so he could work on taking care of himself.

CHAPTER 15.

Religion and Spirituality

THE PERKS AND PERILS OF RELIGION

Thales, a Greek philosopher, would have definitely gotten himself in trouble with modern evangelicals Pat Robertson, Ted Haggard, or Jim Dobson. He proposed the outrageous idea of a non-religious explanation of the cosmos. This was 500 years before a Jewish preacher walked the desert of historical Palestine galvanizing people to change their ways, inspiring a movement more than 2 billion of us call our own to this day (strictly speaking the honor of inspiration should go to Paul, but that detail is often not mentioned in religious history class). I have met many people who find solace and structure in prayer and religion, and if you are one of them, you can skip this section.

There is evidence that prayer and distant healing might have a positive effect on health and healing (Astin et al., 2000, Roe et al., 2015). I don't want to wade too deep into the scientific debate on the topic, but as usual the devil is in the details, or, more scientifically speaking, on the continuum of human existence. If you want to delve into the subject, at least differentiate the studies by who is doing the praying— you, the patient, or others around you? Do you as a patient benefit from praying, or do you benefit from others praying for you? Quite a distinction here.

Religion and spirituality can add richness to peoples' lives, and I can easily honor the importance. But I don't want the agnostics and atheists among you to despair as I also witness the distress that spirituality and religion can cause despite its beneficial effects on many. This was definitely true for Shelley and Karen.

Shelley had always done the right thing. She had a deep connection to God that helped her guide her life as a teacher and human being. She is one of the people with the most integrity I have ever met. She inspired her students and co-teachers and always lent a hand to friends. Her dedication did not spare her from cancer.

She underwent grueling treatments bravely. After a long time of rehabilitation, she was looking forward to returning to work. The treatment had left her with limitations that required accommodations at work, and her employer, lacking Shelly's integrity, let her go despite her many years of service. To make matters worse, within a brief period of time, Shelley also lost both her parents. And estrangement with the remaining family followed.

Shelley's world came unglued. She desperately tried to hold on to her belief system. She talked with God to find meaning in what was happening to her. She also looked to God for answers to her situation and guidance on how to go forward. None of it helped to solve the day-to-day problems. Shelley's life transformed from reasonable comfort to near poverty. Stripped of her ability to earn a living, she needed to learn to depend on others. She bravely swallowed her pride and piece by piece surrendered her independence while still maintaining her pride and integrity. She applied for Social Security disability, scaled back her lifestyle, and moved in with an acquaintance.

Karen, a lovely Catholic patient whom I introduced while discussing how people will often try to attribute causes to their cancer, was convinced that an abortion earlier in her life had been the cause of her multiple myeloma. God had punished her for her sin. Let's look at her question, "Why is God punishing me with cancer?" For Karen's situation, this question evoked quite a bit of distress. On a physiological level, the question equated to a thought produced by Karen's brain that had a slew of unpleasant emotions attached. For Karen it was difficult to imagine that the question was just a thought and not her actual reality.

Neither Shelley's nor Karen's cancer had anything to do with God but simply poor luck. Karen did not cause her cancer by having an abortion, and

Shelley's cancer had no meaning. It simply sucked. Neither woman had done anything wrong. But both experiences illustrate principles that we encountered earlier in the book.

One is the human desire for understanding and causality. While Karen "knew" that a "sin" had caused the cancer, Shelley represented the other side of the same coin. Since she had lived impeccably, the cause of her illness stayed mysteriously hidden, and she despaired in speculations about what she had done wrong in God's eyes. Both were mentally preoccupied with the distress-causing thoughts of causality instead of the health-promoting acceptance of uncertainty.

It is true that spirituality and yearning for meaning increase for people when confronted with an illness, but that does not mean that the cancer itself has meaning. Dealing with cancer makes us more aware of our mortality and stimulates us to want to add more meaning and purpose to life. Cancer becomes the trigger to expand meaning.

And with Shelley's and Karen's stories, we also revisit the point that it is not belief systems per se that get you in trouble. The trouble stems from the clash of your belief system with reality. Shelley's belief that a devout life equates to a healthy life clashed with the reality of getting sick. She also got disappointed in her belief that all Christians were good people with integrity, like herself. Being laid off from her religious school while sick was not compatible with her belief about the goodness in Christians. This conflict between belief and reality caused considerable distress. Instead of understanding the mechanics of her thinking and how it affected her well-being, Shelley got stuck in despair about her relationship with God.

I tell Shelley's and Karen's stories not to discourage you from or judge you for seeking spirituality and religion, but I do encourage a pause if the pursuit causes you distress. Consider that the health-promoting effects of spiritualty only seem to work if you believe in a benevolent God. Research now shows that patients who believe that God does not love them have detrimental changes in their immune system (Ironson et al., 2011). That in itself would not be a problem, but according to a survey by Baylor University published in 2006, only 23 percent of people in the U.S. believe in a benevolent God (Bader et al., 2006). Five percent are atheist, and the rest believe in either an authoritarian, angry, or distant God.

We don't even have to argue whether God exists (which the vast majority of Americans do); if your spiritual or religious beliefs are inducing distress, your health will suffer. The crucial point is how the body differentiates negative and positive thoughts (no matter their veracity) and how those thoughts affect the body. We are right back to our core premise of Mr. Baldwin's experience with himself and the world.

As a physician, I had to approach both women's situation without challenging their belief systems, regardless of my own views. Karen had already been on a path of separating from her childhood religious beliefs before she was diagnosed with cancer. In extensive discussions, we settled that the question, "Why is god punishing me with cancer?" simply was a sentence and not a fact. However, since Karen had thought that sentence so many times, it had established itself in her brain. You remember from Jill Smolowe's book *Four Funerals and a Wedding*, which I mentioned in the section on **Nagging Thoughts and the Principle of Rigidity** from **Chapter 4**, that thoughts have a tendency to groove. In Karen's case, that long-ago established nerve fibers generating the thought "Why is God punishing me with cancer?" still existed, even when Karen recognized the thought as not representing her reality anymore. Gradually she was able to decrease the frequency and intensity of thinking the thought, and as her brain fibers shrank, so did the associated emotions of guilt and shame.

SOULS AND SPIRITS

I casually used the word "soul" at the beginning of the book. I don't really know what soul is. But since many people seem to have a clear sense, I felt free to use it in a way I thought was suitable. I assume it roughly belongs in the category "spirituality." Some entity that is more than just the product of our cells. Some entity that is beyond reasoning and will create heated debates about its nature. One supposed proof I was given for the existence of same came during a conversation about the transitioning process from life to death. My sparring partner was sure that the mysterious thing that disappears in the transition from life to death is the soul. Having been present during many deaths, I have often wondered exactly what happens in that moment. While I can see how someone would use that word in that context, to me it is not a convincing argument for the existence of the soul.

"Spirituality" is another word that gets my brain gears going. When I once raised the question about what "spirit" is, my discussion partner attributed my lack of "understanding" to my Germanic language background. I do know, however, that the German word "Geist" kicks the same brain gears of questioning curiosity in motion. This is not a language problem. I am not sure what that makes me, but the closest I can come in language is a *naturalist*—a person who explains the world and humans with laws of nature.

Having said that, being a naturalist does not prevent me from conversing and connecting with others of a different worldview. If anything it makes for lively conversation learning from each other. My task is to connect on the plane my patient lives on and to assist with change in a desired direction. Allow me to mention a book that you might find helpful if this subject engages you, Kate Bowler's *Everything Happens for a Reason*. Kate Bowler, who wrote her dissertation on the prosperity gospel, was confronted with her beliefs after she was diagnosed with cancer. Her writing movingly describes how she oscillated between her religious beliefs and her critical thinking and balanced doubt and hope all at once. Readers might find her discourses helpful. Ultimately it boils down to finding acceptance and peace with wherever we are on the spiritual and religious continuum to get through cancer as balanced as possible.

CHAPTER 16.

Living with Illness

People don't like to hear the word *cancer*, but the terms *metastatic cancer* or *incurable cancer* are even more evocative. As I had discussed in **Chapter 11** in the section on **Stage and Type of Cancer**, the word *cancer* covers such a broad range of conditions that using it is tricky in itself. I had used the analogy that saying "I have cancer" is similar to saying "I own a method of transportation" or "I work in a hotel." The term is not differentiated enough to adequately express what's going on with you medically (or emotionally for that matter). It covers the whole spectrum from "I had a cancerous mole removed" to "I have three months to live." That generality and simplification open the door to misinterpretations and assumptions that cause confusion. What you need to remember is there are versions of cancer you can live with for many years, even if you are not cured. I am not just talking about precursors of illness as is common in blood or skin cancer but ongoing and even metastatic illness. Sometimes a houseguest is here to stay.

EXERCISES

If you are in that category of "metastatic illness," I want you to pause for a moment and consider an image that allows you not to see yourself as an entity dominated by cancer. Can you see yourself as a huge meadow of flowers, every flower representing your trillions of cells? Yes, there are some plants on that meadow that are dried up or ill, but they don't negate the beauty of the meadow as a whole. While you have to address the fact that some of your cells need treatment— the same way you might weed your garden—I want you to remember that you are made up of trillions of cells, and even though some of your cells are cancer cells, there are many, many more healthy cells than unhealthy ones.

Let's do an exercise that is very similar to **Our Second Awareness Exercise** in **Chapter 1** that allows you to remember how many healthy cells you have and that these cells can help you stay as healthy as possible and as balanced as possible while you deal with your cancer.

In the earlier awareness exercise, I had you focus on your healthy cells and how they produce thoughts, emotions, and body sensations. Taking a look at the non-healthy cells can be frightening. Pause for a moment and sense if you are ready to reflect on non-healthy cells. Nothing wrong with wanting to skip it! But if want to jump into the—figuratively speaking—ice water, start by scanning your body for an assessment of healthy versus unhealthy cells. Is your attention drawn toward cells with cancer? If you are still uncomfortable, you can repeat the healthy cell exercise as a warm-up.

Notice how the warm-up exercise makes you feel. Do you feel more tense? Do you feel more relaxed? Has an emotion shifted? Or has a body sensation changed? Do your thoughts reveal information you can learn from?

If you feel ready for the "bad" cell exercise, I want you to conjure up an image of a cancer cell. Again you can either let an image emerge from your imagination or take a look at a book or online what such a cell might look like. Do you feel nervous thinking and feeling about the cancer cells, or can you look at these cells as the ones that your treatment is eliminating or at least keeping at bay? What imagery comes up to destroy those cells? You can visualize crushing or vaporizing them. Use an image that you mentally create or one that comes up spontaneously.

An important point to remember: I don't want you to hear me encourage you to exclusively use imagery techniques for the elimination of cancer cells but view them as part of your arsenal of tools. Notice how your emotions and your body shift when you take mental control of your own situation. If the exercise lifts your mood, lightens your body, and creates positive thoughts, you are in business. Always use your breath in between reflections and experiences to help your body balance.

TREATMENT WITH PSYCHEDELIC MEDICINES

I wasn't quite sure where to place this section as I am convinced that treatments that enhance non-ordinary states of consciousness can help at any phase or stage of cancer. Some people use the term altered state of consciousness, but I prefer non-ordinary. It refers to a state that's different from what we ordinarily spend most of our waking time in. You can enter a non-ordinary state of consciousness with hypnosis, certain types of breath, or treatment with psychedelic medication. The technique might not matter with respect to your personal experience, but I do want to discuss psychedelic medication in particular given their historical importance and recent resurrection. They have a long tradition in aiding cancer patients. Since clinical trials with cancer patient have been mostly conducted in advanced stages of cancer, I am mentioning the treatment in this chapter. Exploring and processing existential concerns is a fundamental core of any kind of supportive therapy for cancer, particularly advanced cancer. Patients are not just concerned about death and meaning but also minimizing suffering and fear of isolation (Spiegel & Kogon, 2022).

Our society is fortunately getting closer to the FDA approving such treatment outside of clinical trials because of successes in populations with cancer (Griffiths et al., 2016, Ross et al., 2016) and Posttraumatic Stress Disorder (Mitchell et al., 2021).

Plant-based assistance has been part of human culture for millennia, experiencing waves of support or suppression depending on the societal and political flavor of the day. We are currently seeing a resurrection of solid treatments for cancer patients that had already been successfully studied in the 1950s and 1960s before being suppressed in the 1970s and then reentering scientific study in the 1990s. Particularly since the publication of Michael Pollan's book *How to Change Your Mind*, the knowledge has jumped out of the academic institutions into mainstream culture. If this is something that interests you, find the latest trials you might qualify for at www.clinicaltrials.gov.

QUANTITY VERSUS QUALITY OF LIFE

I have already touched on this idea in the section on **Competing Needs** in **Chapter 9** when discussing your interactions with your doctor on the topic. While the question of quantity versus quality of life matters for all phases and stages of illness, it becomes most prominent towards the end of life.

Morton had to make an important decision whether to agree to yet another surgery, not with the aim to cure his cancer but to hopefully buy him some time. He was tired from his many years of treatment and was contemplating to discontinue them. In an honest conversation with his physician about his quality of life after surgery, the verdict was that Morton would at best spend his days in a chair reading, but that his proactive lifestyle of exercise, shopping, and cooking for himself was over. It took him little time to decide that this was not satisfying. His adult daughter, a working mother of two, who was listening in immediately protested, calling her father selfish. How could he not consider enjoying a life sitting in a chair being a joy to his family?

This exchange illustrates yet again the principle of competing needs. Morton, having endured many years of treatment, pain, and increasing physical limitations opted for quality of life, while his daughter—overwhelmed with her busy life—idealized a life being housebound, longing for more rest herself. The two were able to communicate their differences, but it required an intervention with a professional to recognize their different needs with respect to quality and quantity of life. When they understood how the other felt, they were open to discuss practical options both could accept.

TOWARD THE END

The focus of this book is not hospice care, but many of the mechanisms explained in this book apply to end of life as well. As I mentioned early on, there is plenty of good literature for this part of life. For those interested, I will recommend several books. As I mentioned in the beginning, patients have been dying from cancer for millennia, so the available literature is broad. What's new is surviving cancer and living with cancer. *Not the Last Goodbye* by David Servan-Schreiber, *Marrow* by Elizabeth Lesser, *Before I go* by Paul Kalanithi, *Four Funerals and a Wedding* by Jill Smolowe, *Dying Well* and *The Four*

Things That Matter Most by Ira Byock, *The Last Lecture* by Randy Pausch and *Enjoy Every Sandwich* by Lee Lipsenthal are just a few of many accounts that deal with end of life from different perspectives. They are also books about love, compassion, grief, family, relationship, and resilience. All experiences closely associated with death and dying.

Often patients develop a sense that the end nears, and consequently a strong need to turn inward emerges. This can be challenging for family and friends, who want to enjoy as much time as possible with their loved one. It is difficult not to experience the turning inward as rejection. But remember the bell curve and competing needs.

Figure 25 shows that the patient is moving away from enjoying closeness toward the end of their life, and the family members might be doing the opposite, feeling an increased need for closeness. They might not start out in different places but will head in opposite directions with changing needs. When the distance on the bell curve grows, there is a good chance for sadness, conflict, and disappointment for everyone involved.

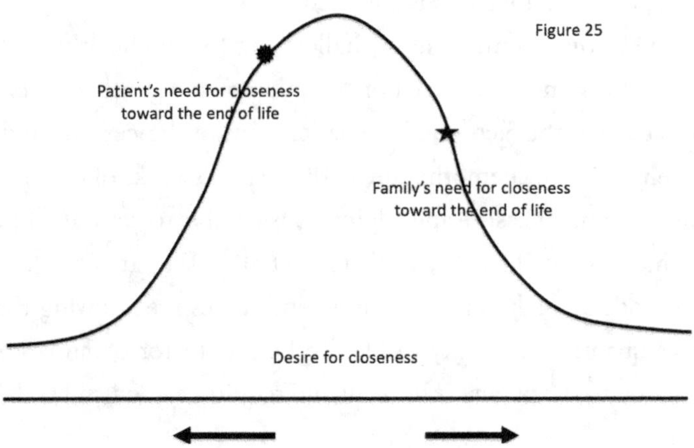

Figure 25

You have seen this figure before as it represents a core concept of this book. Acknowledging and reconciling differences. The bigger the difference on the bell curve, the higher the chance at having to pay close attention to avoid disappointment and disagreement.

But the opposite can be true. As patients are getting closer to death, they can be unrealistic in their expectations of life expectancy and the treatments to get them there. They are so attached to life that they are not realistic about their actual circumstances. Erwin had been in the prime of his life as a civil engineer when he was diagnosed with metastatic cancer. He fought his illness bravely, but his decline was gradual and eventually became obvious. His cognitive ability decreased, he had issues with balance and ultimately could not take care of himself.

He kept inquiring about the latest treatments, medication, and rehab facilities, even when it was apparent to everybody that the end was near. He also had an important identity as a provider, and one of the last things he said was that he was concerned that his wife would not be able to survive without him, even though she was fiercely independent and autonomous all her life. Erwin's concern to fight was a reflection of his identity as a provider. Another patient, Sonia, also fought to the last day of her life to get the most aggressive treatments. Yet another patient, Peter, chose a procedure that had a 1 percent chance of extending his life by a year. He survived the procedure but shortly after collapsed in his father's arms and died.

These situations are incredibly challenging for the healthcare team, as well as the patients and their loved ones. An open and gentle conversation is necessary to declare the facts and help patients make choices. Around 10 percent of patients receive chemotherapy in the last two weeks of life, despite not being a life extending measure and adding considerable toxicity and low quality of life (Anshushaug et al., 2015, Wilkerson et al., 2021). It is tempting to go into action mode and administer an intervention despite knowing that it will not improve quantity or quality of life. To be the doctor or nurse to deliver this information to the patient is difficult and requires a good and collaborative relationship.

In this phase of life, it is particularly important not to confuse distress with mental illness. While the literature is not clear-cut, there is evidence that antidepressants in patients with advanced cancer but no mental health diagnosis are often not helpful (Lloyd-Williams et al., 2013).

Talking in metaphors can be more helpful than presenting hard facts.

Lisa was at the end of her life and knew it. At the beginning of her illness, she had expressed a wish to visit her home country. However, when her illness did not allow for to travel, we started a mental journey visiting her childhood home. She could vividly describe the details of her bedroom and the items that had been comforting in her childhood. In our conversations, we rearranged Lisa's bedroom to make it suitable for her current situation. Even though we weren't physically there, it seemed to comfort her. Around that time, she started to slowly drift in and out of consciousness and died shortly after.

Nora, a very dignified lady who was diagnosed with pancreatic cancer, used metaphors of her own. One day she started talking about sunsets. She meticulously described the shades and colors at the different stages of the sun setting. She also described how she saw herself slowly walk towards the sun setting. We both knew that she was talking about her own death. During our conversations, we actually never mentioned the word death but always referred to different ways of walking towards the sun.

A hospice nurse who spends her days with the dying summarized it poignantly: "I never see anyone in here who cares about money or what they have accomplished in life. It only matters how they connected to others. That's what they want to talk about." Cancer cuts across income and wealth. It is an equalizer. You can buy fancier treatment, but you cannot buy well-being. That process happens from within.

While it is true that a majority of people, even towards the end of life, behave in their own particular way, what matters is that there are vast differences between us. As I've said before, we are all unique and fit somewhere on the bell curve of our respective differences. We have to stay open and in the moment to be able to capture what matters. As we have reached the end of this book, I want to emphasize a statement I started it with. The same way you want targeted precision medicine for your body, you also want it for your soul. Coming towards the end of your life doesn't mean it has to be full of despair; it can in fact have serenity in it.

And sometimes the end isn't the end after all. Patients have many motivations to live, and parents particularly do not want to leave young children. Remember Manuel the teacher who struggled balancing his professional identity with his health? When first diagnosed, he was given two years to live. He lived for six, and I believe that wanting to see and support his teenage son growing into adulthood had something to do with it.

And even when the end is truly near, be open for anything. Very touching things can happen. With the end coming predictably close, Martin decided he did not want to saddle his emotionally savvy but tax illiterate wife with having to file taxes right after his death. He pulled it off, working hard with a heart rate of 35/min and constantly weak and short of breath. He filed taxes on April 15th and left his body behind on April 30th. This one hits particularly close to home as Martin happens to have been my husband of twenty-five years. His last grand gesture has changed me. His dedication, devotion, and commitment are with me most days as a reminder to focus on what matters. Marty, I love you.

I want to close this book with a quote from one of our former presidents, George H. W. Bush. I have found this quote helpful over the years (even though I would have never voted for him). The quote serves all of us as a model for all phases of life and from all walks of life, no matter what life presents us with.

> **Tell the truth. Don't blame people. Be strong. Try hard.**
> **Forgive. Stay the course.**

REFERENCES

BOOKS

Achor, Shawn. (2010). *The happiness advantage: the seven principles of positive psychology that fuel success and performance at work* (1st ed.). New York: Broadway Books.

Begley, Sharon. (2007). *Train your mind, change your brain: how a new science reveals our extraordinary potential to transform ourselves*. New York: Ballantine Books.

Barrett, Lisa F. (2017). *How emotions are made: The secret life of the brain*. Boston: Houghton Mifflin Harcourt.

Bowler, Kate. (2019). *Everything Happens for a Reason: And Other Lies I've Loved* Random House Publishing Group.

Byock, Ira. (1997). *Dying Well: The Prospect for Growth at the End of Life*. Thorndike Press.

Cahalan, Susannah. (2019). *The Great Pretender.* New York, Boston: Grand Central Publishing.

Damasio, Antonio R. (1994). *Descartes' error: emotion, reason, and the human brain*. New York: Putnam.

David, Susan. (2016). *Emotional Agility: Get Unstuck, Embrace Change, and Thrive in Work and Life*. New York: Avery/Penguin Random House.

Doidge, Norman. (2015). *The brain's way of healing: remarkable discoveries and recoveries from the frontiers of neuroplasticity*. Viking, 1st edition.

Dittrich, Luke. (2016) *Patient H.M. : a story of memory, madness and family secrets* (First edition. ed.). Random House.

Duckworth, Angela. (2016) *Grit: The Power and Passion of Perseverance*. Scribner.

Dweck, Carol. (2007). *Mindset*. Ballantine.

Eagleman, David. (2011). *Incognito: The Secret Lives of the Brain*, 1st American ed. New York: Pantheon Books.

Epictetus. *Discourses 3-4. Fragments. The Encheiridion*. Translated by W. A. Oldfather. Loeb Classical Library 218. Cambridge, MA: Harvard University Press, 1928.

Gallagher, Winifred. (2009). *Rapt : attention and the focused life*. New York: Penguin Press.

Gladwell, Malcolm. (2005). *Blink : the power of thinking without thinking* (1st ed.). New York: Little, Brown and Co.

Gladwell, Malcolm. (2008). *Outliers : the story of success* (1st ed.). New York: Little, Brown and Co.

Gray, John. (1992). *Men are from Mars, Women are from Venus*. New York: Harper Collins.

Hanh, Thich N. (1976). *The Miracle of Mindfulness: A manual of meditation*. Beacon Press.

Hanson, R., & Mendius, R. (2009). *Buddha's brain: The practical neuroscience of happiness, love & wisdom*. New Harbinger Publications.

Harris, Dan. (2014). *10% happier : how I tamed the voice in my head, reduced stress without losing my edge, and found self-help that actually works : a true story*. Harper Collins.

Hawkes, Joyce Whiteley. (2006). *Cell-level healing: the bridge from soul to cell* (1st ed.). New York: Atria Books.

Jung, Carl Gustav. (1953). *Collected works. Vol. 12. Psychology and alchemy*. Pantheon Books.

Kalanithi, Paul. (2016). *When breath becomes air*. New York: Random House.

Kesler, Shelli. (2013). *Improving Cognitive Function After Cancer.* South Carolina: CreateSpace Publishing.

Langer, Ellen J. (2009). *Counter clockwise : mindful health and the power of possibility* (1st ed.). New York: Ballantine Books.

Lesser, Elizabeth. (2016). *Marrow : a story of love, loss & what matters most*. New York: Harper Collins.

Levitin, Daniel J. (2014). *The Organized Mind : Thinking Straight in the Age of Information Overload*. New York : Penguin Random House.

Lipsenthal, Lee. (2011). *Enjoy Every Sandwich: Living Each Day as If It Were Your Last* (1st ed.). Harmony.

Lipton, Bruce H. (2005). *The biology of belief: unleashing the power of consciousness, matter and miracles* (1st ed.). Santa Rosa, CA: Mountain of Love/Elite Books.

Lutz, Tom. (1999). *Crying: The Natural and Cultural History of Tears*. New York: W.W. Norton&Company.

McGonigal, Kelly. (2015). *The Upside of Stress.* New York: Penguin Random House.

Nestor, James. (2020). *Breath*. London, England: Penguin Life.

Newport, Cal. (2016). *Deep work: rules for focused success in a distracted world* (First Edition. ed.). New York, Boston: Grand Central Publishing.

Norem, Julie K. (2001). *The positive power of negative thinking: using defensive pessimism to manage anxiety and perform at your peak*. Cambridge, MA: Basic Books.

Pausch, Randy., & Zaslow, Jeffrey. (2008). *The Last Lecture* (1st ed.). Hyperion.

Pert, Candace B. (1997). *Molecules of emotion : why you feel the way you feel.* New York, NY: Scribner.

Pollan, Michael. (2019). *How to Change Your Mind: What the New Science of Psychedelics Teaches Us About Consciousness, Dying, Addiction, Depression, and Transcendence*. Penguine Press.

Riggs, Nina. (2018). *The Bright Hour: A Memoir of Living and Dying* (Reprint ed.). Simon & Schuster.

Rosenberg, Marshall. (2005). *Nonviolent Communication*. Encinitas, CA: PuddleDancer.

Salzberg, Sharon. (2013). *Real happiness at work: meditations for accomplishment, achievement, and peace*. New York: Workman Publishing Company, Inc.

Sapolsky, Robert M. (2004). *Why Zebras Don't Get Ulcers*, 3rd ed. New York: Times Books.

Seppälä, Emma. (2016). *The Happiness Track*. HarperCollins, New York.

Servan-Schreiber, David. (2008). *Anticancer-A new way of life*. New York: Viking.

Servan-Schreiber, David, & Gauthier, Ursula. (2011). *Not the last goodbye : on life, death, healing, and cancer*. New York: Viking.

Shawn, Allen. (2007). *Wish I could be there : notes from a phobic life*. New York: Viking.

Siegel, Daniel J. (2010). *Mindsight : the new science of personal transformation* (1st ed.). New York: Bantam Books.

Smith, Daniel. (2012). *Monkey mind: A Memoir of Anxiety*. New York: Simon and Schuster.

Smolowe, Jill. (2014). *Four Funerals and a Wedding. Resilience in a Time of Grief.* She Writes Press, Berkeley.

Solomon, Andrew. (2001). *The Noonday Demon: An Atlas of Depression*. New-York: Scribner.

Spiegel, David & Kogon, Manuela. (2022). *Supportive-Expressive Group Therapy and the Terminally Ill* In Chochinov HM, Breitbart W (Eds) *Handbook of Psychiatry in Palliative Medicine*, 3rd Edition. Oxford University Press.

Tolle, Eckhart. (1999). *The Power of now*. Namaste.

Van der Kolk, Bessel A. (2014). *The body keeps the score : brain, mind, and body in the healing of trauma*. Viking.

Waal, Frans. (2016). *Are we smart enough to know how smart animals are?* W. W. Norton & Company, New York.

Walker, Matthew. (2018). *Why we sleep*. Penguin Books.

Whippman, Ruth. (2016). *America the anxious : how our pursuit of happiness is creating a nation of nervous wrecks* (First U.S. edition. ed.) New York: St. Martin's Press.

Wolynn, Mark. (2016). *It didn't start with you : how inherited family trauma shapes who we are and how to end the cycle*. New York: Viking.

JOURNAL ARTICLES

Andrews-Hanna, J. R. (2012). The brain's default network and its adaptive role in internal mentation. *Neuroscientist, 18*(3), 251-270. doi: 10.1177/1073858411403316

Anshushaug, M., Gynnild, M. A., Kaasa, S., Kvikstad, A., & Grønberg, B. H. (2015). Characterization of patients receiving palliative chemo- and radiotherapy during end of life at a regional cancer center in Norway. *Acta oncologica (Stockholm, Sweden)*, *54*(3), 395–402.
https://doi.org/10.3109/0284186X.2014.948061

Assous, A., Borghini, A., Levi-Rueff, M., Rittori, G., Rousselot-Pailley, B., Gosme, C., Zigante, F., Golse, B., Falissard, B., & Robel, L. (2018). Children with mixed developmental language disorder have more insecure patterns of attachment. *BMC psychology*, *6*(1), 54. https://doi.org/10.1186/s40359-018-0268-6

Astin, J. A., Harkness, E., & Ernst, E. (2000). The efficacy of "distant healing": a systematic review of randomized trials. *Annals of internal medicine*, *132*(11), 903–910. https://doi.org/10.7326/0003-4819-132-11-200006060-00009

Bray, V. J., Dhillon, H. M., Bell, M. L., Kabourakis, M., Fiero, M. H., Yip, D., Boyle, F., Price, M. A., & Vardy, J. L. (2017). Evaluation of a Web-Based Cognitive Rehabilitation Program in Cancer Survivors Reporting Cognitive Symptoms After Chemotherapy. *Journal of clinical oncology : official journal of the American Society of Clinical Oncology*, *35*(2), 217–225. https://doi.org/10.1200/JCO.2016.67.8201

Beardslee, W. R., Versage, E. M., & Gladstone, T. R. (1998). Children of affectively ill parents: a review of the past 10 years. *Journal of the American Academy of Child and Adolescent Psychiatry*, *37*(11), 1134–1141. https://doi.org/10.1097/00004583-199811000-00012

Benarroch E. E. (2020). Physiology and Pathophysiology of the Autonomic Nervous System. *Continuum (Minneapolis, Minn.)*, *26*(1), 12–24. https://doi.org/10.1212/CON.0000000000000817

Berman, M. G., Kross, E., Krpan, K. M., Askren, M. K., Burson, A., Deldin, P. J., Kaplan, S., Sherdell, L., Gotlib, I., H., Jonides, J. (2012). Interacting with nature improves cognition and affect for individuals with depression. *J Affect Disord*, *140*(3), 300-305. doi: 10.1016/j.jad.2012.03.012

Campbell, H. S., Sanson-Fisher, R., Turner, D., Hayward, L., Wang, X. S., & Taylor-Brown, J. (2010). Psychometric properties of cancer survivors' unmet needs survey. *Supportive care in cancer : official journal of the Multinational Association of Supportive Care in Cancer*, *19*(2), 221–230. https://doi.org/10.1007/s00520-009-0806-0

Carlson, L.E., Waller, A., Mitchell, A.J. (2012). Screening for distress and unmet needs in patients with cancer: review and recommendations. *J Clin*

Oncol 30 (11): 1160-77.

Caspi, A., Roberts, B. W., & Shiner, R. L. (2005). Personality development: stability and change. *Annu Rev Psychol, 56*, 453-484. doi:10.1146/annurev.psych.55.090902.141913

Cimprich, B., & Ronis, D. L. (2003). An environmental intervention to restore attention in women with newly diagnosed breast cancer. *Cancer Nurs, 26*(4), 284-292; quiz 293-284.

Cohen, S., Doyle, W. J., Turner, R. B., Alper, C. M., & Skoner, D. P. (2003). Emotional style and susceptibility to the common cold. *Psychosom Med, 65*(4), 652-657.

Collet, C., Vernet-Maury, E., Delhomme, G., & Dittmar, A. (1997). Autonomic nervous system response patterns specificity to basic emotions. *Journal of the autonomic nervous system, 62*(1-2), 45–57. https://doi.org/10.1016/s0165-1838(96)00108-7

Collaborative Group on Hormonal Factors in Breast Cancer. (1997). Breast cancer and hormone replacement therapy: collaborative reanalysis of data from 51 epidemiological studies of 52,705 women with breast cancer and 108,411 women without breast cancer. *Lancet, 350*(9084), 1047-1059.

Costa-Requena, G., Ballester Arnal, R., & Gil, F. (2013). Perceived social support in Spanish cancer outpatients with psychiatric disorder. *Stress and health : journal of the International Society for the Investigation of Stress, 29*(5), 421–426. https://doi.org/10.1002/smi.2488

Crum, A. J., & Langer, E. J. (2007). Mind-set matters: exercise and the placebo effect. *Psychol Sci, 18*(2), 165-171. doi: 10.1111/j.1467-9280.2007.01867.x

De Couck, M., Caers, R., Musch, L., Fliegauf, J., Giangreco, A., & Gidron,

Y. (2019). How breathing can help you make better decisions: Two studies on the effects of breathing patterns on heart rate variability and decision-making in business cases. *International Journal of Psychophysiology : official journal of the International Organization of Psychophysiology*, *139*, 1–9. https://doi.org/10.1016/j.ijpsycho.2019.02.011

Deepak K. K. (2019). Meditation induces physical relaxation and enhances cognition: A perplexing paradox. *Progress in brain research*, *244*, 85–99. https://doi.org/10.1016/bs.pbr.2018.10.030

Dement W. C. (1997). The perils of drowsy driving. *The New England Journal of Medicine*, *337*(11), 783–784. https://doi.org/10.1056/NEJM199709113371111

Derogatis, L. R., Morrow, G. R., Fetting, J., Penman, D., Piasetsky, S., Schmale, A. M., Henrichs, M., & Carnicke, C. L., Jr (1983). The prevalence of psychiatric disorders among cancer patients. *JAMA*, *249*(6), 751–757. https://doi.org/10.1001/jama.249.6.751

Ebede, C. C., Jang, Y., & Escalante, C. P. (2017). Cancer-Related Fatigue in Cancer Survivorship. *The Medical clinics of North America*, *101*(6), 1085–1097. https://doi.org/10.1016/j.mcna.2017.06.007

Ekman, P. (1992). Are there basic emotions? *Psychol Rev*, *99*(3), 550-553.

Forte, G., Favieri, F., & Casagrande, M. (2019). Heart Rate Variability and Cognitive Function: A Systematic Review. *Frontiers in neuroscience*, *13*, 710. https://doi.org/10.3389/fnins.2019.00710

Fredrickson, B. L., & Losada, M. F. (2005). Positive affect and the complex dynamics of human flourishing. *The American psychologist*, *60*(7), 678–686. https://doi.org/10.1037/0003-066X.60.7.678

Friedman, H. L., & Brown, N. (2018). Implications of Debunking the "Critical Positivity Ratio" for Humanistic Psychology: Introduction to Special Issue. *Journal of humanistic psychology*, *58*(3), 239–261. https://doi.org/10.1177/0022167818762227

Giese-Davis, J., Collie, K., Rancourt, K. M., Neri, E., Kraemer, H. C., & Spiegel, D. (2011). Decrease in depression symptoms is associated with longer survival in patients with metastatic breast cancer: a secondary analysis. *Journal of clinical oncology : official journal of the American Society of Clinical Oncology*, *29*(4), 413–420. https://doi.org/10.1200/JCO.2010.28.4455

Gottman, J.M., Levenson, R.W. (2002). A two-factor model for predicting when a couple will divorce: exploratory analyses using 14-year longitudinal data. *Fam Process*, *41*(1):83-96.

Griffiths, R. R., Johnson, M. W., Carducci, M. A., Umbricht, A., Richards, W. A., Richards, B. D., Cosimano, M. P., & Klinedinst, M. A. (2016). Psilocybin produces substantial and sustained decreases in depression and anxiety in patients with life-threatening cancer: A randomized double-blind trial. *Journal of psychopharmacology (Oxford, England)*, *30*(12), 1181–1197. ttps://doi.org/10.1177/0269881116675513

Hossain, J. L., & Shapiro, C. M. (2002). The prevalence, cost implications, and management of sleep disorders: an overview. *Sleep Breath*, *6*(2), 85-102. doi: 10.1007/s11325-002-0085-1

Ironson, G., Stuetzle, R., Ironson, D., Balbin, E., Kremer, H., George, A., Schneiderman, N., Fletcher, M. A. (2011). View of God as benevolent and forgiving or punishing and judgmental predicts HIV disease progression. *J Behav Med*, *34*(6), 414-425. doi: 10.1007/s10865-011-9314-z

Janelsins, M. C., Kesler, S. R., Ahles, T. A., & Morrow, G. R. (2014). Prevalence, mechanisms, and management of cancer-related cognitive impairment.

Int Rev Psychiatry, *26*(1), 102-113. doi: 10.3109/09540261.2013.864260

Jang, E. H., Byun, S., Park, M. S., & Sohn, J. H. (2019). Reliability of Physiological Responses Induced by Basic Emotions: A Pilot Study. *Journal of Physiological Anthropology*, *38*(1), 15. https://doi.org/10.1186/s40101-019-0209-y

Kaplan, S., & Berman, M. G. (2010). Directed Attention as a Common Resource for Executive Functioning and Self-Regulation. *Perspect Psychol Sci*, *5*(1), 43-57. doi: 10.1177/1745691609356784

Kim S.H., Kim Y.H., Kim H.J. (2015) Laughter and Stress Relief in Cancer Patients: A Pilot Study. *Evid Based Complement Alternat Med.*
doi: 10.1155/2015/864739.

Kreibig, S. D. (2010). Autonomic nervous system activity in emotion: a review. *Biol Psychol*, *84*(3), 394-421. doi: 10.1016/j.biopsycho.2010.03.010

Lange, M., Joly, F., Vardy, J., Ahles, T., Dubois, M., Tron, L., Winocur, G., De Ruiter, M. B., & Castel, H. (2019). Cancer-related cognitive impairment: an update on state of the art, detection, and management strategies in cancer survivors. *Annals of oncology : official journal of the European Society for Medical Oncology*, *30*(12), 1925–1940. https://doi.org/10.1093/annonc/mdz410

LeDoux, J. E. (2000). Emotion circuits in the brain. *Annu Rev Neurosci*, *23*, 155-184. doi: 10.1146/annurev.neuro.23.1.155

LeDoux, J. E., & Pine, D. S. (2016). Using Neuroscience to Help Understand Fear and Anxiety: A Two-System Framework. *Am J Psychiatry*, *173*(11), 1083-1093. doi: 10.1176/appi.ajp.2016.16030353

LeDoux, J. E. (2020). Thoughtful feelings. *Current biology : CB*, *30*(11), R619–R623. https://doi.org/10.1016/j.cub.2020.04.012

Joormann, J., Talbot, L., & Gotlib, I. H. (2007). Biased processing of emotional information in girls at risk for depression. *Journal of abnormal psychology*, *116*(1), 135–143. https://doi.org/10.1037/0021-843X.116.1.135

LeMoult, J., Joormann, J., Kircanski, K., & Gotlib, I. H. (2016). Attentional bias training in girls at risk for depression. *Journal of child psychology and psychiatry, and allied disciplines*, *57*(11), 1326–1333. https://doi.org/10.1111/jcpp.12587

Lick, D. J., Cortland, C. I., Johnson, K. L. (2016). The pupils are the windows to sexuality: pupil dilation as a visual cue to others' sexual interest. *Evolution and Human Behavior 37*(2), 117-124, doi: 10.106/j.evolhumbehav.2015.09.004

Lloyd-Williams, M., Payne, S., Reeve, J., & Kolamunnage Dona, R. (2013). Antidepressant medication in patients with advanced cancer—an observational study. *QJM*, *106*(11), 995-1001. doi: 10.1093/qjmed/hct133

Löwel, S., & Singer, W. (1992). Selection of intrinsic horizontal connections in the visual cortex by correlated neuronal activity. *Science*, *255*(5041), 209-212

Lupien, S. J., Maheu, F., Tu, M., Fiocco, A., & Schramek, T. E. (2007). The effects of stress and stress hormones on human cognition: Implications for the field of brain and cognition. *Brain Cogn*, *65*(3), 209-237. doi: 10.1016/j.bandc.2007.02.007

Massie, M. J., & Holland, J. C. (1987). Consultation and liaison issues in cancer care. *Psychiatric medicine*, *5*(4), 343–359.

McCraty, R., Atkinson, M., Tomasino, D., Bradley, R.T., (2009). The coherent heart heart-brain interactions, psychophysiological coherence, and the emergence of system-wide order. *Integral Review* 5(2), 10-115

McCraty, Rollin & Shaffer, Fredric. (2015). Heart Rate Variability: New Perspectives on Physiological Mechanisms, Assessment of Self-regulatory Capacity, and Health risk. *Global Advances in Health and Medicine* : 4(1), 46-61

McIntosh, A. M., Hall, L. S., Zeng, Y., Adams, M. J., Gibson, J., Wigmore, E., Hagenaars, S. P., Davies, G., Fernandez-Pujals, A. M., Campbell, A. I., Clarke, T. K., Hayward, C., Haley, C. S., Porteous, D. J., Deary, I. J., Smith, D. J., Nicholl, B. I., Hinds, D.A., Jones, A. V., Scollen, S., Meng, W., Smith, B. H.Hocking, L. J. (2016). Genetic and Environmental Risk for Chronic Pain and the Contribution of Risk Variants for Major Depressive Disorder: A Family-Based Mixed-Model Analysis. *PLoS Med*, *13*(8), e1002090. doi: 10.1371/journal.pmed.1002090

Mitchell, A. J., Ferguson, D. W., Gill, J., Paul, J., & Symonds, P. (2013). Depression and anxiety in long-term cancer survivors compared with spouses and healthy controls: a systematic review and meta-analysis. *Lancet Oncol*, *14*(8), 721-732. doi: 10.1016/S1470-2045(13)70244-4

Mitchell, J. M., Bogenschutz, M., Lilienstein, A., Harrison, C., Kleiman, S., Parker-Guilbert, K., Ot'alora G, M., Garas, W., Paleos, C., Gorman, I., Nicholas, C., Mithoefer, M., Carlin, S., Poulter, B., Mithoefer, A., Quevedo, S., Wells, G., Klaire, S. S., van der Kolk, B., Tzarfaty, K., … Doblin, R. (2021). MDMA-assisted therapy for severe PTSD: a randomized, double-blind, placebo-controlled phase 3 study. *Nature medicine*, 27(6), 1025–1033. https://doi.org/10.1038/s41591-021-01336-3

Mora-Ripoll R. (2010). The therapeutic value of laughter in medicine. *Alternative therapies in health and medicine*, *16*(6), 56–64.

Nahin, R. L., Boineau, R., Khalsa, P. S., Stussman, B. J., & Weber, W. J. (2016). Evidence-Based Evaluation of Complementary Health Approaches for Pain Management in the United States. *Mayo Clinic proceedings*, *91*(9), 1292–1306. https://doi.org/10.1016/j.mayocp.2016.06.007

Ordaz, S. J., LeMoult, J., Colich, N. L., Prasad, G., Pollak, M., Popolizio, M., Price, A., Greicius, M., Gotlib, I. H. (2017). Ruminative brooding is associated with salience network coherence in early pubertal youth. *Soc Cogn Affect Neurosci*, *12*(2), 298-310. doi: 10.1093/scan/nsw133

Palesh, O. G., Mustian, K. M., Peppone, L. J., Janelsins, M., Sprod, L. K., Kesler, S., Innominato, P. F., Roth, T., Manber, R., Heckler, C., Fiscella, K., & Morrow, G. R. (2012). Impact of paroxetine on sleep problems in 426 cancer patients receiving chemotherapy: a trial from the University of Rochester Cancer Center Community Clinical Oncology Program. *Sleep medicine*, *13*(9), 1184–1190. https://doi.org/10.1016/j.sleep.2012.06.001

Räikkönen, K., Matthews, K. A., Flory, J. D., Owens, J. F., & Gump, B. B. (1999). Effects of optimism, pessimism, and trait anxiety on ambulatory blood pressure and mood during everyday life. *Journal of personality and social psychology*, *76*(1), 104–113. https://doi.org/10.1037//0022-3514.76.1.104

Roe, C. A., Sonnex, C., & Roxburgh, E. C. (2015). Two meta-analyses of noncontact healing studies. *Explore (New York, N.Y.)*, *11*(1), 11–23. https://doi.org/10.1016/j.explore.2014.10.001

Ross, S., Bossis, A., Guss, J., Agin-Liebes, G., Malone, T., Cohen, B., Mennenga, S. E., Belser, A., Kalliontzi, K., Babb, J., Su, Z., Corby, P., & Schmidt, B. L. (2016). Rapid and sustained symptom reduction following psilocybin treatment for anxiety and depression in patients with life-threatening cancer: a randomized controlled trial. *Journal of psychopharmacology (Oxford, England)*, *30*(12), 1165–1180. https://doi.org/10.1177/0269881116675512

Sarris, J., & Byrne, G. J. (2011). A systematic review of insomnia and complementary medicine. *Sleep medicine reviews*, *15*(2), 99–106. https://doi.org/10.1016/j.smrv.2010.04.001

Scheier, M. F., Swanson, J. D., Barlow, M. A., Greenhouse, J. B., Wrosch, C., & Tindle, H. A. (2021). Optimism versus pessimism as predictors of physical health: A comprehensive reanalysis of dispositional optimism research. *The American psychologist*, *76*(3), 529–548. https://doi.org/10.1037/amp0000666

Schreier, A. M., Johnson, L. A., Vohra, N. A., Muzaffar, M., & Kyle, B. (2019). Post-Treatment Symptoms of Pain, Anxiety, Sleep Disturbance, and Fatigue in Breast Cancer Survivors. *Pain management nursing : official journal of the American Society of Pain Management Nurses*, *20*(2), 146–151. https://doi.org/10.1016/j.pmn.2018.09.005

Seligman, M. E., & Maier, S. F. (1967). Failure to escape traumatic shock. *J Exp Psychol*, *74*(1), 1-9.

Shelby, R. A., Golden-Kreutz, D. M., & Andersen, B. L. (2008). PTSD diagnoses, subsyndromal symptoms, and comorbidities contribute to impairments for breast cancer survivors. *J Trauma Stress*, *21*(2), 165-172. doi: 10.1002/jts.20316

Shields, G. S., Sazma, M. A., & Yonelinas, A. P. (2016). The effects of acute stress on core executive functions: A meta-analysis and comparison with cortisol. *Neurosci Biobehav Rev*, *68*, 651-668. doi: 10.1016/j.neubiorev.2016.06.038

Szkodny, L. E., & Newman, M. G. (2019). Delineating Characteristics of Maladaptive Repetitive Thought: Development and Preliminary Validation of the Perseverative Cognitions Questionnaire. *Assessment*, *26*(6), 1084–1104. https://doi.org/10.1177/1073191117698753

Szabó, M. & Lovibond, P.F. (2002) The cognitive content of naturally occurring worry episodes. *Cognitive Therapy and Research* (2002) 26(2): 167-177

Szabó, M., Lovibond, P. F. (2006). Worry episodes and perceived problem solving: A diary-based approach. *Anxiety Stress and Coping*, 19(2), 175-187

Temel, J. S., Greer, J. A., Muzikansky, A., Gallagher, E. R., Admane, S., Jackson, V. A., Dahlin, C. M., Blinderman, C. D., Jacobsen, J., Pirl, W. F., Billings, J. A.Lynch, T. J. (2010). Early palliative care for patients with metastatic non-small-cell lung cancer. *N Engl J Med*, *363*(8), 733-742.
doi: 10.1056/NEJMoa1000678

Ulrich, R. S. (1984). View through a window may influence recovery from surgery. *Science*, *224*(4647), 420-421.

Veenstra, L., Schneider, I. K., & Koole, S. L. (2016). Embodied mood regulation: the impact of body posture on mood recovery, negative thoughts, and mood-congruent recall. *Cogn Emot*, 1-16.
doi: 10.1080/02699931.2016.1225003

Walker M. P. (2009). The role of sleep in cognition and emotion. *Annals of the New York Academy of Sciences*, *1156*, 168–197. https://doi.org/10.1111/j.1749-6632.2009.04416.x

Wefel, J. S., Kesler, S. R., Noll, K. R., & Schagen, S. B. (2015). Clinical characteristics, pathophysiology, and management of noncentral nervous system cancer-related cognitive impairment in adults. *CA Cancer J Clin*, *65*(2), 123-138. doi: 10.3322/caac.21258

Wentzensen, N., & O'Brien, K. M. (2021). Talc, body powder, and ovarian cancer: A summary of the epidemiologic evidence. *Gynecologic oncology*, *163*(1), 199–208. https://doi.org/10.1016/j.ygyno.2021.07.032

Wilkerson, D. H., Santos, J. L., Tan, X., & Gomez, T. H. (2021). Too Much Too Late? Chemotherapy Administration at the End of Life: A Retrospective Observational Study. *The American journal of hospice & palliative care*, *38*(10), 1182–1188. https://doi.org/10.1177/1049909120966619

Wilkes, C., Kydd, R., Sagar, M., & Broadbent, E. (2017). Upright posture improves affect and fatigue in people with depressive symptoms. *Journal of behavior therapy and experimental psychiatry*, *54*, 143–149. https://doi.org/10.1016/j.jbtep.2016.07.015

Yang, Y., Cao, S., Shields, G. S., Teng, Z., & Liu, Y. (2017). The relationships between rumination and core executive functions: A meta-analysis. *Depression and anxiety*, *34*(1), 37–50. https://doi.org/10.1002/da.22539

Zaccaro, A., Piarulli, A., Laurino, M., Garbella, E., Menicucci, D., Neri, B., & Gemignani, A. (2018). How Breath-Control Can Change Your Life: A Systematic Review on Psycho-Physiological Correlates of Slow Breathing. *Frontiers in human neuroscience*, *12*, 353. https://doi.org/10.3389/fnhum.2018.00353

Zhang, Y., Padmanabhan, A., Gross, J. J., & Menon, V. (2019). Development of Human Emotion Circuits Investigated Using a Big-Data Analytic Approach: Stability, Reliability, and Robustness. *The Journal of neuroscience: the official journal of the Society for Neuroscience*, *39*(36), 7155–7172.

Zhou, H. X., Chen, X., Shen, Y. Q., Li, L., Chen, N. X., Zhu, Z. C., Castellanos, F. X., & Yan, C. G. (2020). Rumination and the default mode network: Meta-analysis of brain imaging studies and implications for depression. *NeuroImage*, *206*, 116287. https://doi.org/10.1016/j.neuroimage.2019.116287

OTHER SOURCES

Bader, Christopher, Dougherty, Kevin, Froese, Paul Johnson F., Byron, Mencken, Carson Park, Jerry Z., Stark, Rodney (2006) https://www.baylor.edu/baylorreligionsurvey/doc.php/288937.pdf

Dushek, Jennie (2016) An emerging view of evolution is informing cancer research https://med.stanford.edu/news/all-news/2016/08/an-emerging-view-of-evolution-is-informing-cancer-research.html

Grierson, Bruce, New York Times, October 22, 2014. What if Age Is Nothing but a Mind-Set? https://www.nytimes.com/2014/10/26/magazine/what-if-age-is-nothing-but-a-mind-set.html

Jaouad, Suleika, New York Times, March 17, 2015. Out of the Woods, Into the Dark, http://nyti.ms/1GeTwAQ

Hoffman, Jan, New York Times, November 2, 2015. Good news about worrying. New York Times, https://well.blogs.nytimes.com/2015/11/02/while-waiting-for-test-results-worrying-may-help-in-the-long-run/

Killion, Ann San Francisco Chronicle March 19, 2019. Cal swimming alum Nathan Adrian reveals his bout with testicular cancer. https://www.sfchronicle.com/sports/annkillion/article/Cal-swimming-alum-Nathan-Adrian-reveals-his-bout-13702002.php

Kazziha, Khaled, SFGate, September 26, 2016. Some elephants learning to avoid dangerous areas. https://www.sfgate.com/world/article/Some-elephants-learning-to-avoid-dangerous-areas-9289306.php

Kost, Ryan, San Francisco Chronicle, November 21, 2021. The reality is sinking in: There will be no COVID closure https://www.sfchronicle.com/bayarea/article/With-no-clear-end-in-sight-to-pandemic-Bay-Area-16636292.php

Kourlas, Gia, New York Times, October 22, 2014. A choreographer retrains his body to move again. https://www.nytimes.com/2022/03/03/arts/dance/ronald-k-brown-recovery.html

LaRosa, John, November 2013, https://www.slideshare.net/jonlar/the-us-self-improvement-market

Semnani, Neda, Washington Post, September 23, 2016, A Harvard psychol-

ogist explains why forcing positive thinking won't make you happy
https://www.washingtonpost.com/news/inspired-life/wp/2016/09/23/forcing-positive-thinking-wont-make-you-happy-says-this-harvard-psychologist/

Winn, Steven, San Francisco Chronicle, October 13, 2021, Kenneth Baker, longtime Chronicle arts critic, dies at 75
https://datebook.sfchronicle.com/art-exhibits/kenneth-baker-longtime-chronicle-arts-critic-dead-at-75

INDEX

www.ingramcontent.com/pod-product-compliance
Lightning Source LLC
LaVergne TN
LVHW011631200926
848484LV00011B/2549/J